KEGEL

EXERCISE FOR MEN

BEGINNERS

A compressive guide to build up your pelvic floor muscle triumph over erectile dysfunction and take charge of your health sex life

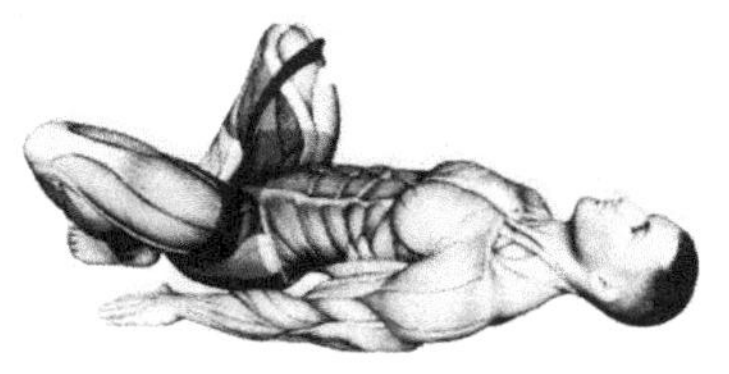

MATTHEW BREWER

Table of Content

Introduction..6

Chapter 1: Unveiling the Powerhouse Beneath Understanding Your Pelvic Floor...............9

What are Pelvic Floor Muscles and Why Are They Important for Men?.................................... 9

Unveiling the Benefits of Strong Pelvic Floor Muscles for Men's Health..............................11

Sexual Performance and Enhanced Pleasure........14

Improved Bladder Control and Reduced Urinary Leakage.. 17

Potential Role in Erectile Dysfunction Management...20

Overall Core Strength and Improved Posture...22

Chapter 2: Finding Your Foundation: Mastering the Art of Kegel Exercises....................................26

Discovering Your Pelvic Floor Muscles: Techniques and Tips.. 26

The "Urine Stop" Technique............................29

Alternative Techniques for Identifying Pelvic Floor Muscles...31

Performing Kegel Exercises Effectively: Technique Makes Perfect...34

Supine (Lying Down) Position..........................37

Seated Position..39

Standing Position...42

The Art of Diaphragmatic Breathing: Coordinating Breath with Kegels.....................45

Exercise Variations for a Well-Rounded Kegel Routine.. 47

Marches (Toe Taps)...................................... 50

Speedy Flick Kegels...................................... 52

Heel Slides..55

Happy Baby Pose....................................... 58

Lying Down... 61

Sitting..64

Side Lying... 67

Hands and Knees...................................... 70

Squatting...73

Single-Leg Bridge...................................... 76

(For Advanced Individuals:) Kegel with Ball Squeeze...80

Chapter 3: Building a Sustainable Routine: Frequency, Consistency, and the Power of Progress. 84

How Often Should You Practice Kegel Exercises?.84

How Many Kegel Exercises Should a Man Do Per Day?... 86

Building a Sustainable Kegel Routine: Tips for Consistency... 88

Chapter 4: Fueling Your Core: Optimizing Your Diet for Kegel Success....................................92

Understanding the Link Between Diet and Pelvic Floor Health... 92

Foods to Embrace for a Stronger Core...................94

Fruits and Vegetables: Packed with Essential Nutrients... 97

Whole Grains: Providing Sustained Energy..........103

Healthy Fats: Supporting Hormone Balance........ 107

Chapter 5: Foods to Minimize: Keeping Your Core

Clean..112

Processed Foods and Added Sugars: The Inflammatory Culprits.. 112

Excessive Saturated and Trans Fats: Hindering Blood Flow.. 116

Excessive Caffeine and Alcohol: Potential Disruptors 120

Chapter 6: Beyond the Basics: Exploring Advanced Techniques for Experienced Men.............................125

Fast Kegels vs. Slow Kegels: Tailoring Your Routine for Specific Goals...125

Slow Kegels: Building Strength and Endurance... 129

Leveling Up Your Kegel Game: Advanced Techniques for Experienced Men......................... 133

Biofeedback Training: Receiving Real-Time Feedback on Your Technique.............................. 141

Chapter 7: Kegel Exercises and Erectile Dysfunction: A Potential Ally...................................... 146

Understanding Erectile Dysfunction and Its Causes... 146

The Potential Role of Kegel Exercises in Erectile Dysfunction Management...................................... 152

Strengthening Pelvic Floor Muscles for Improved Blood Flow... 158

Enhancing Sexual Stamina and Performance...... 164

Important Considerations: When to Consult a Doctor Regarding Erectile Dysfunction............................. 169

Chapter 8: Building a Stronger You: Exercises to Complement Your Kegel Routine...........................175

Leg Lunges: Engaging Multiple Muscle Groups... 175

Plank Variations: Building Core Strength and

Stability.. 180

Squats: Targeting Lower Body Strength and Core
Activation... 187

**Chapter 9: Maintaining Momentum: Overcoming
Challenges and Staying Motivated......................... 193**

Overcoming Challenges and Staying Motivated with
Your Kegel Routine.. 193

Celebrating Progress and Recognizing
Achievements.. 199

Incorporating Kegel Activities into Your Regular
routine for Long haul Advantages........................204

**Chapter 10: The Power Within: Conclusion and
Taking Charge of Your Health...............................209**

Disclaimer

Introduction

How does a man know if he is doing Kegels correctly?

Hey guys, let's talk about Kegels. Presently, I understand what you may be thinking - another exhausting work-out daily routine. But, trust me, this is unique. It's tied in with assuming command, about rediscovering a strength you never realized you had, and eventually, about feeling like the best version of yourself.

But here's the thing: when I initially began with Kegels, I was totally lost. Without a doubt, I read instructions online, and I even watched videos, yet entirely nothing clicked. Could it be said that I was crushing the right muscles? Could it be said that I was treating them terribly? It was baffling, no doubt. Imagine investing this energy and not getting results in light of the fact that your strategy is off. That is the reason I needed to compose this book - to be the assistance I really wanted in those days.

Consider this your guide to Kegel authority. We'll break it down step by step, so you can be certain you're in good shape. Everything really revolves around feeling the association, that inconspicuous fixing profound inside.

No more mystery, not any more contemplating whether you're getting things done well. We should open the power inside and take your wellbeing and prosperity to an unheard of level.

All in all, would you say you are prepared to feel the distinction? How about we make a plunge and find the key to dominating those Kegels!

Can men do Kegels while sitting?

So guys, we should discuss something the vast majority of us presumably wouldn't even for a second consider raising at the rec center, among companions, or even with a specialist - Kegels. It can feel abnormal, isn't that so? However, trust me, I get it. As a man myself, I went through years dubiously mindful of Kegels yet never truly plunged into what they were or how to do them. We should simply say, my insight came from a problematic web look and a ton of deception.

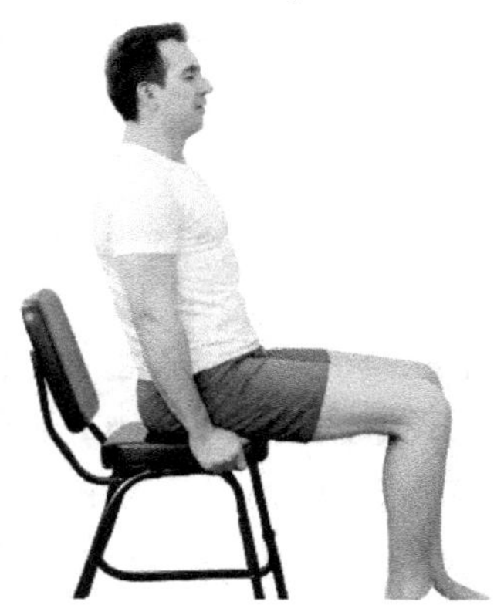

In any case, stop and think for a minute, after at last going all in and figuring out how to do Kegels appropriately, try to keep your hat on - it's been a distinct advantage. Not only for my room life (in spite of the fact that, can we just be real for a moment, that is an unequivocal advantage!), yet for my general wellbeing and prosperity as well.

Presently, you may ponder, "Could you at any point even do Kegels while sitting?" The response is totally! As a matter of fact, plunking down can be an incredible method for learning the strategy prior to continuing on toward different positions. Consider this - Kegels aren't some enormous, conspicuous development. They're unpretentious, and that really makes them so viable.

Thus, ditch the humiliation and go along with me on this excursion. We will separate Kegels for fledglings, bit by bit, while you're easily chilling on that seat. No extravagant hardware is required, just you and a readiness to assume command over your wellbeing. We should open the capability of your pelvic floor muscles and see what sort of astounding outcomes we can accomplish together. Trust me, you will love it!

Chapter 1: Unveiling the Powerhouse Beneath Understanding Your Pelvic Floor

What are Pelvic Floor Muscles and Why Are They Important for Men?

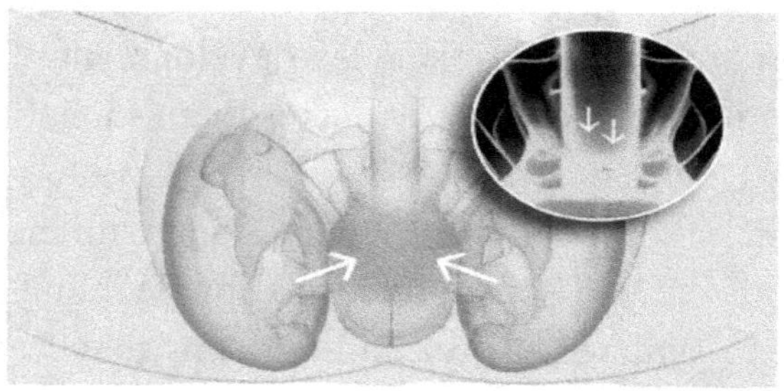

Can we just be real, guys, we don't precisely invest a great deal of energy contemplating our pelvic floor muscles. Not a subject comes up at the exercise center or over lagers with the pals. Yet, trust me, these secret legends down there merit some serious consideration.

Why? Since they gigantically affect our wellbeing and prosperity in manners we probably won't understand.

Recall the last time you laughed so hard your sides hurt, or perhaps you sniffled excessively powerfully and... indeed, how about we simply say there was an unwanted shock. Those, my companions, are indications of a frail pelvic floor. These muscles behave like a lounger, supporting your bladder, guts, and that immeasurably significant pipes down there. At the point when they're solid, they keep everything set up, yet when they're powerless, things can get somewhat... cracked.

In any case, it's not just about trying not to humiliate circumstances (despite the fact that, can we just be look at things objectively, who needs to manage that?). Solid pelvic floor muscles assume a key part in our sexual presentation as well. Envision attempting to hit a homer with an unbalanced bat - that is the very thing sex can feel like with frail pelvic floor muscles. You probably won't have the control or endurance you want.

Here is the uplifting news: very much like some other muscle, your pelvic floor can be reinforced! It could sound unusual from the get go, however with a touch of training, you can turn into your very own expert center. Furthermore, accept me, the advantages merit the work. You'll insight:

Further developed bladder control: Not any more unforeseen releases, in any event, when you chuckle or wheeze. Certainty, anybody?

Upgraded sexual execution: More grounded erections, better control, and more endurance. Well that is something to think of home about!

Generally center strength: A solid pelvic floor interfaces with your center, prompting better stance and an all the more remarkable constitution. Stand tall, honorable men!

Anyway, would you say you are prepared to assume responsibility for your wellbeing and open the power inside? We should plunge into the following part, where we'll investigate precisely how to find these subtle pelvic floor muscles and get everything rolling on your excursion to a more grounded, better you.

Unveiling the Benefits of Strong Pelvic Floor Muscles for Men's Health

---

Let's face it, guys, we don't frequently discuss our "down there" wellbeing. It's a place where there is secret, in some cases covered in a bit (or a ton) of humiliation. In any case, listen to this, there's a secret power place settled underneath the surface, an organization of muscles called the pelvic floor, and try to keep your hat on, getting to realize these folks can be a unique advantage.

Presently, I'm not discussing some for the time being hero change. In any case, throughout recent months, since I began zeroing in on fortifying my pelvic floor, I've seen a few genuine, substantial advantages that have really shocked me (positively!). Here's the reason you, old buddy, ought to think about going along with me on this excursion:

1. Room Euphoria: Can we just be real, this is presumably the principal thing that strikes a chord when we discuss men's wellbeing, correct? Indeed, solid pelvic floor muscles can be your clear-cut advantage for a really fulfilling sexual coexistence. They assist with blood stream down there, which can prompt firmer erections and, we should simply say, a more "present" feeling during closeness. Envision those taken looks across the room having a totally different significance - an importance powered by certainty and control.

2. Cracked Business? That's it: Fellows, we've all been there. Perhaps that surprising wheeze surprised you, or you snickered excessively hard at a pal's joke. Spillage occurs, yet it ought not be a standard event. Solid pelvic floor muscles behave like a characteristic dam, holding everything set up when you want it most. Not any more abnormal sodden spots or that steady concern in your sub-conscience. Envision the opportunity of partaking in life's little astonishments unafraid.

3. Past the Room: The advantages of serious areas of strength for a story go far past your sexual coexistence. These muscles are the groundwork of your center, supporting your spine and stance. Recollect that pestering lower back torment you get in the wake of a monotonous day? Solid pelvic floor muscles can assist with reducing that by taking a portion of the pressure away from you. Envision feeling taller, and more grounded, with a recently discovered trust in your walk.

4. Assuming Command: There's something enabling about assuming responsibility for your own wellbeing. By zeroing in on your pelvic floor, you're adopting a proactive strategy to your prosperity. It's as of now not a uninvolved onlooker in your life, it's a functioning member. Envision the fulfillment of realizing you're putting resources into your future wellbeing, each Kegel practice in turn.

These are only a portion of the advantages I've encountered, and trust me, it's an excursion worth taking.

Presently, the uplifting news is, that you don't require extravagant gear or a rec center enrollment to begin. In the following part, we'll dig into the universe of Kegel works out, a basic yet strong method for opening the secret capability of your pelvic floor. How about we do this together, folks. Now is the right time to assume back command and experience the advantages of serious areas of strength for a, from the room to the meeting room and in the middle between.

Sexual Performance and Enhanced Pleasure

Let's be honest, guys. We as a whole need to be certain lions in the room, the ones who amaze our accomplices and need more. However, in some cases, indeed, life tosses curves. Stress, weariness, that additional cut of pizza the previous evening - everything can negatively affect our presentation.

But fear not, my kindred heroes! There's an unmistakable advantage concealing underneath the surface, ready to be released: your pelvic floor muscles. Presently, I can read your mind - Kegels? Those sound like something your grandmother does. Be that as it may, trust me, these activities are not even close to exhausting. As a matter of fact, dominating them can be a distinct advantage in the room.

Here's the thing: solid pelvic floor muscles resemble an ensemble guide for your ground floor blend. They control blood stream, sensation, and, we should not neglect, endurance. Also, the most awesome aspect? Reinforcing them is more straightforward than you naturally suspect. I began my Kegel venture a couple of months back, wary however inquisitive. You will scarcely believe, the outcomes have been stunning (straightforwardly!).

Imagine this: you're at the time, things are warming up, and you can feel a flood of control you never knew existed. You can expand the joy, uplift the force, and leave your accomplice dumbfounded. It's a certain help that spills over into each part of your life.

All in all, how would we take advantage of this enchantment? Lock in, in light of the fact that I'm going to make you on a stride by-step manual for Kegel joy:
Tracking down Your Internal Maestro: The initial step is recognizing those subtle pelvic floor muscles. However, imagine yourself halting your pee halfway (don't really do this routinely!). Those muscles you hold are the ones we're later.

The Large Press: Presently, envision you're delicately lifting your lower areas towards your paunch button. That is the Kegel withdrawal. Hold it for a count of three, then unwind for another three. Rehash this multiple times, going for the gold over the course of the day.

The Specialty of Consistency: Like any beneficial thing throughout everyday life, results take time and devotion. Try not to get deterred in the event that you don't feel like a superhuman immediately. Stay with it, and inside half a month, you'll begin seeing a distinction. More grounded erections, expanded control, and the endurance to leave your accomplice asking for more - that is the Kegel sorcery at work.

Remember, this is a journey, not a destination. There will be days when you fail to remember your Kegels, days when life gets insane. Yet, don't thump yourself. Simply jump back on the pony and continue to rehearse. Trust me, your future self (and your partner) will thank you.

So, are you ready to unleash your inner rockstar? It all starts with a simple squeeze. Let's rewrite the script on bedroom performance, together.

Improved Bladder Control and Reduced Urinary Leakage

How about we talk genuinely. Spilling pee. It's not precisely a subject we raise at evening gatherings. Be that as it may, for the majority of us, myself included, it's a disappointing and some of the time humiliating reality. The consistent stress over that unforeseen stream, the frantic race to the restroom, the sensation of vulnerability - it can negatively affect your certainty and personal satisfaction.

Just take my for it, I've been there. Wheezes that transformed into runs, chuckling that transformed into quiet frowns, that consistent desire to "for good measure" myself. It seemed like my body had deceived me, and the dissatisfaction was overpowering. However, here's the uplifting news: I didn't need to live like that until the end of time. There are ways of recovering control, and I'm here to impart my excursion to you, bit by bit, in the expectations it enables you to recover yours.

<u>Stage 1: Recognize and Comprehend</u>

The initial step is recognizing there's an issue. Overlooking it won't make it vanish. However, prior to jumping into arrangements, understanding the "why" behind the breaks is significant. Did labor debilitate your pelvic floor muscles? Could it be said that you are encountering regular hacks or a urinary lot disease? Conversing with your PCP is critical. They can assist with distinguishing the reason and suggest the best strategy.

<u>Stage 2: Embrace the Force of Pelvic Floor Activities</u>

Brace yourself for what I'm about to tell you, these activities could sound entertaining, yet they are champions in camouflage! Envision a lounger holding your bladder, uterus (on the off chance that you have one), and rectum. Those loungers are your pelvic floor muscles. Kegels resemble little weightlifting meetings for these muscles, making them more grounded and better at supporting your organs.

Presently, finding these muscles can be precarious from the start. Envision you're attempting to stop your pee stream halfway (don't really do this consistently!). That fixing sensation? Those are your pelvic floor muscles! Whenever you've recognized them, hold the press for a couple of moments, then unwind. Rehash this multiple times, three times each day. It probably won't feel like much from the beginning, yet trust me, consistency is critical!

Stage 3: Way of life Changes for a Release Free Future

There are some way of life changes that can likewise have a major effect. Turn into a bladder criminal investigator! Notice what sets off your holes - is it sure beverages? Fiery food? Lessen or kill those triggers. Likewise, center around bladder preparing. Rather than racing to the restroom at the primary urge, take a stab at hanging on for a couple of moments to expand your bladder limit bit by bit.

Stage 4: Observe Little Triumphs

Keep in mind, recapturing control is an excursion, not an objective. There will be mishaps, days when the holes return. However, don't allow that to put you down! Praise the little triumphs - a whole shopping for food trip without stress, a giggle without a scramble to the restroom. These are indications of progress, and they merit a psychological high-five!

You Are Not Alone

Here is the main thing I believe you should be aware: you are in good company. Urinary spillage is a typical issue, and there is positively no disgrace in looking for help. With the right methodology, you can recover control and carry on with a sure, release free life. Thus, take a full breath, embrace the excursion, and recollect that, you have this!

Potential Role in Erectile Dysfunction Management

See, fellas, can we just be real. Erectile brokenness (ED) - it's a point a large portion of us would prefer to keep away from. It tends to be a genuine disaster for the self image, leaving you feeling baffled, shaky, and perhaps disengaged from your accomplice. Just take my for it, I've been there.

However, consider this: I wasn't prepared to surrender. Sex is an essential piece of a solid relationship, and honestly, it's downright charming! In this way, I began digging, exploring all that I could about ED. There were pills, siphons, peculiar contraptions - a wide range of choices. However at that point I coincidentally found something unforeseen: Kegel works out.

Presently, I'll concede, from the start, I jeered. Crushing a few muscles down there? Truly? Be that as it may, after some persuading (and can we just be real, franticness), I chose to try it out. What did I need to lose?

Try to keep your hat on, it wasn't similar to flipping a switch. It required some investment, some training, and a ton of "Am I doing this right?" minutes. Be that as it may, gradually, continuously, things began to change. I saw a distinction in my erections - they became firmer, more maintained. Sex with my accomplice turned out to be more pleasant and more satisfying for the two of us.

Presently, I'm not saying Kegels are an enchanted shot remedy for ED. Each circumstance is unique, and there could be fundamental clinical reasons having an effect on everything. In any case, stop and think for a minute: they can be an integral asset, and they're totally normal, sans drug, and something you can do completely all alone.

Here is the most outstanding aspect: regardless of whether you're not encountering ED, Kegels are as yet a phenomenal method for reinforcing your pelvic floor, which can prompt better climaxes, further developed bladder control, and, surprisingly, a lift in your general center strength.

Thus, on the off chance that you're interested about Kegels and their capability to further develop your sexual coexistence, here's a bit by bit manual for kick you off:

1. **Tracking down Your Establishment:** We'll discuss how to recognize your pelvic floor muscles - it's more straightforward than you could suspect!
2. **Excelling:** Gain proficiency with the legitimate strategy for performing Kegel works out, including various positions and breathing activities.
3. **Building Consistency:** We'll examine how frequently and for how long you ought to perform Kegels to get results.

Keep in mind, folks, assuming responsibility for your sexual wellbeing is engaging. Make sure to try, find what works for you, and rediscover the flash in your sexual coexistence. obliged.

Things being what they are, would you say you are prepared to release your inward rockstar? Everything begins with a straightforward crush. We should revamp the content on room execution, together.

Overall Core Strength and Improved Posture

You will scarcely believe, I wasn't generally the stance banner kid. My days were spent slouched over a work area, shoulders drooped, lower back a steady hurt. It wasn't simply actually depleting; it destroyed my certainty. I felt undetectable like I was contracting into myself. However at that point, I found the enchantment of center strength and stance improvement, and it's a unique advantage I need to impart to you.

This isn't just about looking great (in spite of the fact that, can we just be look at things objectively, standing tall feels pretty darn fabulous). It's tied in with feeling solid, stimulated, and prepared to take on the world. It's tied in with having the certainty to stroll into a room and own it.

Presently, I understand what you may think: "Center activities sound like torment!" Yet trust me, they don't need to be. We will make this stride by-step, with practices you can do anyplace, whenever.

<u>Stage 1: Grasping Your Center</u>

Consider your center your body's force to be reckoned with. It's not only your abs (however those are significant!), an organization of muscles gets from your lower back right down to your pelvis. These muscles balance out your spine, support your stance, and assist you with moving with power and effortlessness.

Stage 2: Feeling the Fire Touch off - Straightforward Activities for Novices

Here is the magnificence - you don't require extravagant gear! We should begin with some central activities that will get your center terminating:

The Board: This could sound scary, however you can make it happen! Begin your lower arms with your elbows shoulder-width separated. Keep your body in an orderly fashion from head to heels, connecting with your center to hold yourself up. Begin with 30 seconds and progressively increment the hold time as you get more grounded.

Bird Canine: This one's tomfoolery (and trust me, it gets your center working!). On all fours, expand one arm and the contrary leg out straight, keeping your back level. Hold for a couple of moments, then switch sides.

Stage 3: Feeling the Distinction - Stance Flawlessness

Presently, how about we talk act. Envision a string pulling you straight up from the crown of your head. Feel your shoulders loosen up down and away from your ears. Protract your spine and fold your jaw somewhat. This isn't tied in with standing unbending, about finding an agreeable arrangement feels solid and upheld.

<u>**Stage 4: Consistency is Vital**</u>

The way to getting results is consistency. Go for the gold minutes of center activities most days of the week. You'll be flabbergasted at how rapidly you begin feeling the distinction - a freshly discovered strength in your developments, a decrease in back torment, and that quite fulfilling sensation of standing tall.

Keep in mind: This is an excursion, not an objective. There will be days when you want to slump, and days while holding a board feels incomprehensible. In any case, show restraint toward yourself, praise your advancement, and above all, have a good time! You're going to open an unheard of degree of solidarity and certainty. Presently go forward, vanquish the world, and stand tall, old buddy!

Chapter 2: Finding Your Foundation: Mastering the Art of Kegel Exercises

Discovering Your Pelvic Floor Muscles: Techniques and Tips

Can we just be real for a minute, folks, discussing our "down there" isn't generally the most agreeable subject. However, listen to me - there's a secret world underneath the surface, an organization of muscles urgent to our well being and satisfaction, and it's time we shed some light on it. I'm discussing the pelvic floor, and trust me, getting to realize these folks can be a unique advantage.

Presently, I'll tell the truth, whenever I first caught wind of Kegel works out, I envisioned something convoluted, a yogic accomplishment that expected long periods of training of some sort or another. In any case, what I found was quite straightforward, and the advantages? Indeed, how about we simply say they were definitely worth the work.

The way to opening the force of Kegels is finding those tricky pelvic floor muscles. It could sound strange, yet I'm here to direct you through it, bit by bit.

<u>Here's what you'll need:</u>
- **A peaceful, confidential space:** This is tied in with interfacing with your body, and interruptions can be a buzzkill.
- **Comfortable garments:** Relax! Tight jeans or a belt can cause it harder to feel those unobtrusive muscle developments.
- **A receptive outlook:** Neglect any assumptions and embrace the excursion of self-disclosure.

<u>Stage 1: The "Envision You're not kidding" Strategy</u>

OK, this could sound somewhat abnormal, however trust me, it works! Envision you're busy utilizing the bathroom, and unexpectedly, you understand you Truly need to hold it in. That crushing sensation you feel? That is your pelvic floor muscles contracting! Presently, I'm not saying you ought to really stop your stream halfway (not beneficial!), however attempt to reproduce that inclination without including any pipes.

<u>Stage 2: Feeling is Accepting</u>

Since you have an overall thought, rests on your back with your knees twisted and feet level on the floor. Loosen up your stomach and bum - we need no undesirable muscle bunches joining the party. Center around your lower areas. Could you at any point feel a slight fixing sensation when you attempt to duplicate that "holding it in" feeling? That is all there is to it! You've found your pelvic floor muscles!

Stage 3: Elective Methodologies
On the off chance that the "halting pee" strategy isn't doing it for you, no problem! Here are a few different choices:

- **The "Lift" Strategy:** Envision you're attempting to take your reproductive organs off the ground (without really moving your hips). This can assist you with separating the pelvic floor muscles.
- **The Finger Test:** OK, this one's somewhat more personal. Tenderly supplement a perfect finger into your rectum (past the sphincter muscle). At the point when you contract your pelvic floor, you ought to feel a fixing around your finger.

Keep in mind: Don't get deterred in the event that it takes a couple of attempts. It resembles mastering any new expertise - a tiny amount of practice makes a huge difference. Also, the uplifting news? When you find those muscles, you'll be well en route to opening a universe of advantages, both truly and inwardly.

Thus, take a full breath, unwind, and leave on this excursion of self-disclosure. You have this!

The "Urine Stop" Technique

Can we just look at things objectively for a moment, folks, discussing our "first floor" can feel a piece off-kilter, particularly with regards to something as personal as Kegel works out. Yet, trust me, with regards to assuming responsibility for your wellbeing and opening a universe of advantages in the room, Kegels are your unmistakable advantage. What's more, the most vital phase in this excursion is dominating the "pee stop" procedure.

Presently, I can read your mind. Halting halfway? Isn't that terrible for you? While it's not prescribed to make this a normal propensity, the "pee stop" is a phenomenal method for distinguishing those slippery pelvic floor muscles we want to focus with Kegel works out.

Stop and think for a minute, for quite a long time, I felt like I was passing up a great opportunity. My perseverance wasn't what it used to be, and how about we simply say, closeness wasn't really fulfilling. Then, at that point, I coincidentally found Kegels, and try to keep your hat on, it was a distinct advantage. Be that as it may, before I could receive the benefits, I needed to find those darn pelvic floor muscles.

<u>**Here's how you can master the "urine stop" technique:**</u>

Raise a ruckus around town: This is a confidential mission, so snatch a few harmony and calm in the restroom.

- **Unwind and Give up:** Void your bladder however much as could be expected. A more full bladder makes it harder to confine the right muscles.
- **Begin the Stream:** Start to pee as you ordinarily would. Take a full breath and spotlight on the sensation.
- **The Decision time:** Presently comes the key part. Envision you're attempting to keep down a wheeze, however down there. Consider squeezing or crushing something inside to end the stream. Try not to grip your stomach or backside, those are party crashers!
- **Did You Feel It?:** On the off chance that you felt a fixing or lifting sensation around your urethra (the cylinder where pee emerges), congrats! You've recently found your pelvic floor muscles. Hold that inclination briefly, then, at that point, gradually deliver and resume pee.

Presently, here's the genuine truth: It probably won't work totally the initial time. Try not to get deterred!

Unwind, take a couple of full breaths, and attempt once more. Perhaps it takes two attempts, perhaps it takes five. Show restraint toward yourself, this is another expertise you're acquiring.

Keep in mind: Don't regularly practice this during normal pee. We're simply getting this strategy to distinguish the right muscles. Whenever you've gotten the hang of it, you can continue on to legitimate Kegel works out, which are a more controlled method for reinforcing those newly discovered pelvic floor muscles.

The "pee stop" procedure could sound somewhat weird, yet trust me, it's the initial step on an excursion to opening a universe of advantages. More grounded erections, better control, and we should not neglect, the possibility to amaze your accomplice - it's everything reachable. In this way, take a full breath, embrace a little weakness, and prepare to find the power inside!

Alternative Techniques for Identifying Pelvic Floor Muscles

Can we just be real, folks? In some cases the entirety "stop your pee halfway" procedure for finding your pelvic floor muscles feels somewhat... unnatural. Also, can we just be real, the dissatisfaction of crushing and stressing, uncertain on the off chance that you're in any event, focusing on the right region, can be sufficient to make you need to surrender altogether. However, dread not, individual traveler on the way to a more grounded center! There are alternate ways of getting to realize your pelvic floor muscles and accept me, I've attempted them all.

The following are a couple of elective procedures that helped me on my excursion, and they may very well be the ideal fit for you as well:

1. The Hack Test: This one could sound somewhat weird, yet trust me, it works! Take a full breath and afterward let out serious areas of strength for a. As you hack, feel an unpretentious fixing or lifting sensation around your pelvic region. That is your pelvic floor taking care of its business! It could take a couple of attempts, however center around that inward fixing, and you'll be well coming.

2. The Fanciful Lift: This strategy is about representation. Envision you have a lift inside your pelvis. Presently, envision yourself gradually crushing the lift upwards, each floor in turn. Feel for that interior commitment as you "lift" the lift. When you arrive at the highest level, gradually discharge and cut the lift down. This perception can assist you with disconnecting the sensation of your pelvic floor muscles contracting.

3. The Mirror, Mirror on the Wall: Alright, this one doesn't include a real mirror (except if you need to!), however everything revolves around body mindfulness. Rests on your back with your knees twisted and feet align with the floor. Presently, delicately crush your butt as though you're attempting to keep down gas. Search for any unpretentious development in your bum - a slight hold or internal draw. That is your pelvic floor at work!

4. Under pressure: This strategy could take a little practice, yet it tends to be extremely powerful. Delicately embed a perfect finger into your rectum (about an inch or thereabouts). Presently, attempt to crush your finger as though you're attempting to hold it set up. You ought to feel a fixing sensation around your finger - that is your pelvic floor muscles contracting!

Keep in mind, tolerance is vital! It could take a training to distinguish your pelvic floor muscles, and that is entirely OK. Try not to get deterred on the off chance that you don't feel it immediately. Continue to attempt these methods, and in the long run, that's what you'll get "aha!" second. Furthermore, trust me, when you find those slippery muscles, the remainder of your Kegel excursion will be a breeze!

Performing Kegel Exercises Effectively: Technique Makes Perfect

Tune in up, fellas. We all have been there, staring at an article about Kegels, siphoned to assume responsibility for our wellbeing, moreover at that point hit with an unexpected stopping point of disarray. "Situating?" it says. "Prostrate? Situated?" Everything looks like something out of a yoga class, definitely not a way to, indeed, you know, enhance our presentation. However, trust me, my companions, situating is the mysterious handshake to opening the force of Kegels. It's the distinction between feeling like you're getting into thin pants two sizes excessively little and feeling that profound, fulfilling commitment of your pelvic floor muscles.

Presently, I'm no more interesting to abnormal rec center minutes. I've attempted Kegels while adjusting on one leg at the sink (not suggested), and brace yourself for what I'm about to tell you, it wasn't pretty. However, through experimentation (and a ton of giggling at myself), I've found three brilliant situating tips for Kegel novices that will make them feel certain and prepared to overcome:

<u>Tip #1: Finding Your Usual range of familiarity</u>
Consider this your Kegel war room. You need to be loose, engaged, and ready to detach those pelvic floor muscles. Here are your three fundamental choices:

- **The Hero's High position:** Falsehood level on your back, knees twisted, and feet level on the floor. This is an exemplary Kegel position for an explanation - it eases the heat off your spine and permits you to feel the association, as a matter of fact.

- **The Fighter's Rest:** Sitting on a firm seat with your feet level on the foundations ponders as well. Simply ensure your back is straight and your shoulders loose. Envision you're a hero enjoying some time off subsequent to vanquishing a front line (of, all things considered, day to day errands).

- **The Thunderous Applause (Not Actually):** You might do Kegels standing up! Simply ensure your feet are shoulder-width separated and your knees marginally bowed. This position is perfect for cautiously pressing in a couple of Kegels over the course of the day.

Tip #2: Inhale Simple, Inhale Profound

Consider this: pausing your breathing during Kegels is a catastrophe waiting to happen. It worries your entire body, making it harder to seclude those pelvic floor muscles. All things being equal, inhale normally all through the activity. Breathe in profoundly through your nose as you unwind, and breathe out leisurely through your mouth as you contract. Trust me, your muscles will thank you for the oxygen.

Tip #3: Tracking down Your Concentration

Envision you're attempting to get a marble with… indeed, you understand. That is the sort of centered commitment you need with your pelvic floor. Try not to hold your abs, rear end, or thighs - everything revolves around those down-there muscles. It could take a couple of attempts to get its hang however you can definitely relax, with a touch of training, you'll be a Kegel star in the blink of an eye.

Keep in mind, folks, situating isn't tied in with accomplishing some ideal yoga present. It's tied in with finding what feels great and permits you to zero in on the job that needs to be done. Thus, unwind, inhale, and prepare to encounter the force of Kegels!

Supine (Lying Down) Position

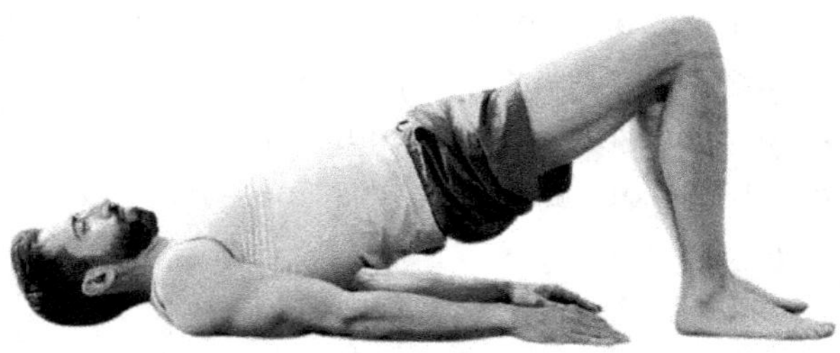

Ok, the prostrate position - for some purposes, it could summon pictures of languid Sundays spent spread on the sofa. In any case, for us folks on the Kegel venture, it's a landmark where we overcome our center and open a universe of stowed away potential. Truly, I've been there, gazing vacantly at the roof, contemplating whether those subtle pelvic floor muscles even existed. However, trust me, this position is your companion, your platform for Kegel significance.

We should separate it, will we? Envision yourself sinking into bed in the wake of a monotonous day. Snatch a comfortable pad, perhaps one you partner with unwinding, and thud yourself down on your back. Legs twisted, knees pointing upwards, feet level on the bedding. This is your beginning stage, a place of solace and weakness. It's where you shed the day's pressure and concentrate internal.

Here is the sorcery: since you're resting, gravity isn't neutralizing you. In contrast to standing or sitting, where your center muscles need to stay at work past 40 hours just to hold you upstanding, here they're loose, fit to be disconnected and designated. It resembles having a quick shortcut for feeling those pelvic floor muscles interestingly.

Presently, shut your eyes. Take a couple of full breaths, feeling your tummy rise and fall with each breathe in and breathe out. This isn't just about Kegels, it's tied in with associating with your body. Envision a warm light filling your center, spreading down to your pelvic floor. This is your power community, and you're going to stir it.

Keep in mind, we as a whole are novices here. Try not to get deterred in the event that you feel nothing immediately. It requires investment and practice, very much like learning another tune on the guitar. However, the magnificence of the prostrate position is that it permits you to analyze, to zero in on the unobtrusive sensations profound inside.

Here is a tip: envision you're attempting to prevent yourself from peeing halfway. Not to really make it happen, obviously, however to get a feeling of that fixing, lifting feeling in your pelvic floor. Presently, hold that inclination for a count of three, then, at that point, discharge it totally. Rehash this multiple times, zeroing in exclusively on that interior commitment.

The recumbent position is your place of refuge, a spot to investigate and find your pelvic floor muscles without judgment. It's where the wizardry works out, where those secret stores of solidarity start to stir. Along these lines, rests, inhale profoundly, and prepare to leave on this intriguing Kegel venture. You have this!

Seated Position

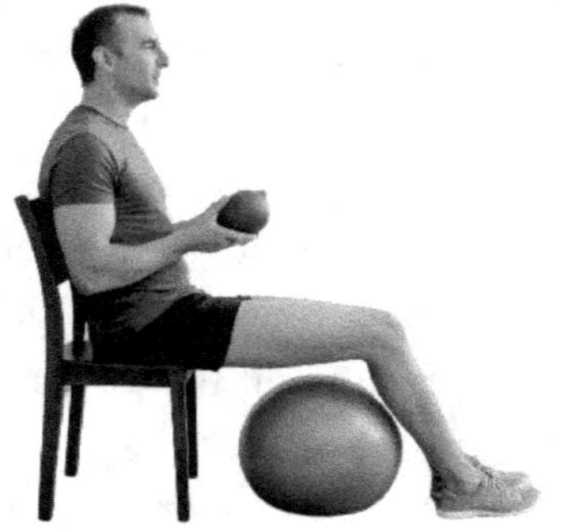

Ok, the situated position. It could appear to be unexceptional from the get go, that seat you thud yourself into each day. However, trust me, with regards to Kegels, acting improves things greatly. It actually tends to be the scaffold among disappointment and that "aha!" second, the distinction between feeling like you're fitting into the pit and really interfacing with those strong pelvic floor muscles.

Presently, I've been on this Kegel venture for some time now, and try to keep your hat on, I've attempted them all - slumped in my office seat, roosted problematically on the edge of the sofa, even endeavored them while folding my legs (enormous no, coincidentally). However, for a novice, the situated position is your brilliant ticket. Here's the reason:

Solace is Vital: Envision this - you're attempting to zero in on these sensitive muscles profound inside, and your back is shouting in fight. Not precisely helpful for an effective Kegel, isn't that so? The situated position permits you to unwind and really tune into your body. Track down a seat with great back help, one that keeps your spine quite straight. Envision a string pulling the crown of your head towards the roof, protracting your neck, and adjusting your stance.

Feet Level on the Floor: This could appear to be a minor detail, however it makes a groundwork of strength. Think about it like structure a house - you really want areas of strength for a preceding you can fabricate anything strong on top. At the point when your feet are level on the floor, it draws in your center muscles quietly, taking some strain away from you and permitting you to zero in on the genuine job that needs to be done - those pelvic floor muscles.

Viewing as Your Middle: Presently comes the tomfoolery part! When you're easily situated with great stance and your feet level, delicately shut your eyes (assuming that you're open to doing as such). Take a full breath through your nose, feeling your tummy extend. As you breathe out leisurely, envision you delicately drawing your gut button inwards, captivating your center. This isn't tied in with sucking in your stomach, yet rather making a delicate enactment of your center muscles.

Furthermore, here's the sorcery: Hold that sensation of a marginally connected center as you endeavor your most memorable Kegel. Envision you're attempting to stop the progression of pee halfway (however kindly, don't really attempt that!). You ought to feel an unobtrusive fixing and lifting sensation profound inside your pelvic floor. Hold for a count of three, then unwind totally for one more count of three. Rehash this multiple times, and that is your most memorable set!

Keep in mind, this is a long distance race, not a run. Try not to get deterred on the off chance that you feel nothing huge from the start. It requires investment and practice to fabricate those muscles. In any case, trust me, with the right stance and a little concentration, you'll feel the force of the situated Kegel in the blink of an eye. Presently go forward and overcome those pelvic floor muscles!

Standing Position

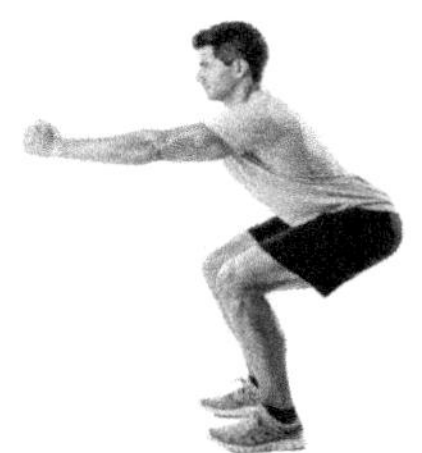

Can we just be real, guys, Kegels can feel a bit... off-kilter from the outset. We're assaulted with pictures of smooth activity machines and extraordinary exercise center exercises, however Kegels? They happen tactfully, in the background. In any case, trust me, there's a sure power in dominating the standing Kegel. It resembles a mysterious handshake with your own body, a method for taking advantage of stowed away holds of solidarity and control.

Presently, I'll concede, I mishandled around with standing Kegels for some time. Envisioning the right muscles wanted to attempt to get smoke. However, consider this: everything without question revolves around pose. Stand tall, old buddy, similar to you're going to meet your legend. Feet shoulder-width separated, toes pointed somewhat internal (think sure, not pigeon-toed). Envision you're hurdling up your center from the back to front, connecting with those profound abs.

Here is the enchanted stunt: take a full breath in, filling your tummy like an inflatable. As you gradually breathe out, imagine yourself tenderly lifting the pelvic floor - those secret muscles down there - without straining your stomach or crushing your glutes. It's an unpretentious sensation, such as holding a solitary drop of water set up. Hold that lift for a count of three, feeling that inward solidness. Then, with a controlled breath, discharge the pressure totally. Unwind, inhale, rehash.

Relax in the event that it takes a couple of attempts. It resembles learning another dance move - somewhat shaky from the beginning, yet with training, you'll track down your musicality. The excellence of the standing Kegel is that you can do it anyplace, whenever. Holding up in line at the supermarket? Ideal chance to crush in a couple of reps (simply don't fault me in the event that the clerk raises an eyebrow!). Stranded in rush hour gridlock? Why not give your pelvic floor a little exercise?

Keep in mind, consistency is critical. Go for the gold arrangements of Kegels over the course of the day, step by step expanding the hold time as you get more grounded. Before long, you'll begin seeing a distinction. Perhaps it's a freshly discovered trust in the room, a more noteworthy feeling of command over your bladder, or just a sensation of being more grounded, more associated with your body.

In this way, stand tall, inhale profoundly, and embrace the force of the standing Kegel. It's a little speculation with enormous settlements, a distinct advantage for a more grounded, better you.

The Art of Diaphragmatic Breathing: Coordinating Breath with Kegels

Ok, diaphragmatic relaxing. It sounds so straightforward, isn't that so? In, out. Simple as pie. Be that as it may, try to keep your hat on, when I initially began integrating this strategy into my Kegel works out, it seemed like attempting to shuffle flaring trimming tools while riding a unicycle. Dissatisfaction doesn't start to cover it.

Yet, stop and think for a minute - when I at long last got a handle on the specialty of diaphragmatic breathing, it turned into a disclosure. It wasn't just about reinforcing my pelvic floor (despite the fact that can we just be real for a minute, that is a really wonderful advantage), it was tied in with rediscovering an association with my own body I never realized I'd lost.

Imagine this: you're worried, shoulders slouched tight, breathing shallow and fast like a cornered creature. That was me. My breaths were these minuscule, overreacted wheezes that scarcely arrived at my chest, not to mention my center. Presently, picture this all things considered: you've recently completed a difficult climb, arrived at the culmination, and are taking in the stunning perspective.

A profound, purging breath fills your tummy, pushing it delicately outwards. A sluggish, fulfilled breath discharges all the strain. That is diaphragmatic relaxing.

It's tied in with saddling the force of your breath and utilizing it to associate with your most profound center muscles. At the point when you do this related to Kegels, it turns into an orchestra - the breath in draws in your stomach, and the breath out agrees with your pelvic floor. It's a strong dance, a discussion between your breath and your body.

What's more, trust me, the advantages go far past the physical. Whenever I first genuinely dominated diaphragmatic breathing during Kegels, a flood of quiet washed over me. It resembled raising a ruckus around the town button on my whole sensory system. Stress that had been stewing underneath the surface began to soften away. My brain felt more clear, more honed. It was like I could at long last inhale once more - in a real sense, yet metaphorically.

In this way, here's my supplication to you, my kindred Kegel confidant: don't underrate the force of diaphragmatic relaxing. It could take some training, a little tolerance, and perhaps a couple of quiet snickers at yourself in the mirror (we've all been there). Be that as it may, when you get it, it turns into an extraordinary device, for your pelvic floor, yet for your general prosperity. It's the unaccounted for part to your Kegel puzzle, the mysterious fixing to opening a more profound feeling of control and quiet. Seriously, it merits the work.

Exercise Variations for a Well-Rounded Kegel Routine

Can we just look at things objectively, folks. At the point when we initially catch wind of Kegels, a couple of things ring a bell: off-kilter quiet, doubtful grins, and perhaps a speedy Google search that leaves you more befuddled than enabled. Be that as it may, trust me, I've been there. I dove carelessly into the universe of Kegels with the best expectations, just to think of myself as addressing on the off chance that I was in any event, doing them right. Perhaps you've envisioned yourself locked away in a room, bending your body into some profane position, just to squeeze...well, something down there.

Be that as it may, here's what I've realized: Kegels don't need to be a task. As a matter of fact, they can be tremendously tomfoolery (and indeed, even somewhat provocative) when you find the assortment that exists! Think about it like structuring your very own Kegel jungle gym - where you can analyze, find what works for you, and eventually, open the genuine capability of your pelvic floor.

Here is a brief look into a portion of my #1 varieties that have taken my Kegel routine from "meh" to "radiant":

The Walk (otherwise known as Toe Taps): Envision yourself driving a victorious triumph march - that is the sort of energy you need to channel here. Fix your pelvic floor muscles with every fanciful "toe tap," feeling that sweet commitment profound inside. It's a phenomenal method for building endurance and control, and can we just be real for a minute, it's downright tomfoolery!

Fast Flick Kegels: Feeling brave? This one's for you. Consider it a fast fire rendition of the exemplary Kegel. Contract your pelvic floor muscles with a progression of fast "flicks," zeroing in on speed as opposed to length. This variety is an extraordinary method for testing your quick jerk muscle strands and work on generally speaking control.

Heel Slides: Envision yourself skimming easily on ice - that is the smooth, controlled feeling you need to accomplish here. Lie on your back with your knees twisted, and gradually slide your heels all over the floor while at the same time getting your pelvic floor muscles. This exercise is an incredible method for developing fortitude and perseverance, leaving you feeling charmingly tested.

Cheerful Child Posture: Recollect those lighthearted long periods of outset? How about we recover a portion of that bliss! Lie on your back, carry your knees to your chest, and snatch your shins (think embracing your knees). Presently, tenderly stone to and fro while pressing your pelvic floor muscles. This perky posture reinforces your center as well as carries a grin to your face - a mutual benefit in my book!

These are only a sample of the numerous varieties you can investigate. The key is to find what feels far better for YOU. Pay attention to your body, try, and don't hesitate for even a moment to get somewhat imaginative! Keep in mind, Kegels are definitely not a one-size-fits-all recommendation. Embrace the excursion, find your interesting way to pelvic floor power, and at last, open a universe of advantages that reach out a long ways past the room.

Marches (Toe Taps)

The Walk, otherwise called Toe Taps, is an incredible Kegel practice variety for fledglings. It's a tomfoolery and connecting method for building control and endurance in your pelvic floor muscles, all while feeling a piece like a victorious pioneer! This is the way to dominate this activity:

Stage 1: Settle in

Find a calm, agreeable space where you can unwind and zero in on your body. You can either lie level on your back with your knees bowed and feet level on the floor, or sit upstanding in a seat with your back straight and feet hip-width separated.

Stage 2: Seclude Your Force to be reckoned with

Envision you're attempting to keep down a surge of pee (however don't really attempt to pee!). This will assist you with drawing in your pelvic floor muscles. Think about them like a lounger supporting your bladder and guts.

Stage 3: Walk Forward!

Presently for the tomfoolery part! Here comes the walk:

- **Fix:** Press your pelvic floor muscles as though you're lifting that interior lounger. Hold briefly - envision this as your "walking foot" descending.
- **Unwind:** Totally discharge your pelvic floor muscles, allowing the lounger delicately to get back to its beginning position. Consider this your foot lifting back up.

Stage 4: Track down Your Mood

Rehash steps 3a and 3b in a consistent, musical movement, imitating the sensation of walking. Go for the gold crushes (about 1 second each) with complete in the middle between. Begin with 10 reiterations and bit by bit increment as you settle in.

- **Favorable to Tip:** Envision yourself driving a celebratory triumph march! Channel that sensation of force and control as you play out your Kegels.
- **Reward Tip:** Inhale regularly all through the activity. Try not to pause your breathing or grip your stomach, rear end, or thighs.

Keep in mind: Consistency is critical! Mean to perform Walks (Toe Taps) a few times each day, steadily expanding the quantity of reiterations as you develop fortitude and control. You'll be shocked at how rapidly this basic activity can turn into a tomfoolery and enable a piece of your day to day everyday practice.

Speedy Flick Kegels

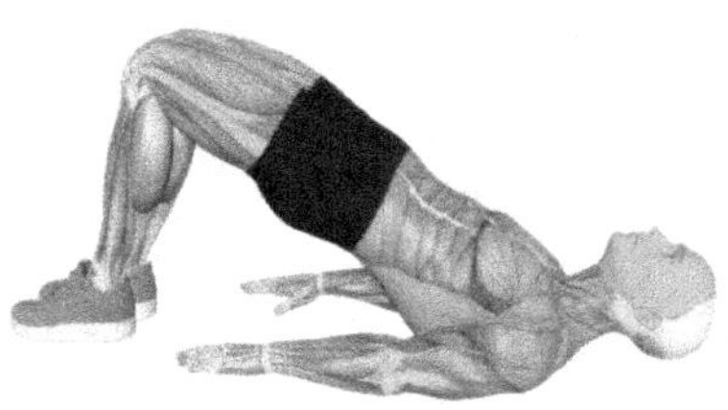

The exemplary Kegel practice gets significantly more energizing with the presentation of Fast Flick Kegels! This variety is about quick compressions and deliveries, testing your pelvic floor muscles in another way. Sit back and relax, regardless of whether you're a finished novice, you can dominate this strategy with these straightforward advances:

Stage 1: Tracking down Your Concentration
Before you hop into speedy flicks, it's vital to know about your pelvic floor muscles. Envision you're attempting to stop your pee stream halfway (don't really do this consistently!). The muscles you use for that are your pelvic floor muscles.

Stage 2: Settle in

Speedy Flick Kegels should be possible in different positions, so find one that feels good and permits you to disengage your pelvic floor muscles. The following are three well known choices:

- **Resting:** This is an incredible beginning position. Lie on your back with your knees bowed and feet level on the floor.
- **Sitting:** Sit upstanding in a seat with your back straight and feet level on the ground.
- **Standing:** Stand with your feet shoulder-width separated and loosen up your shoulders.

Stage 3: Connect with and Delivery (Quick!)

Presently comes the tomfoolery part! This is the way to play out a Fast Flick Kegel:

- **Breathe in:** Take a full breath through your nose.
- **Lock in:** As you breathe out, immediately contract your pelvic floor muscles. Consider it a quick crush, similar to a little clench hand holding and delivering. Go for the gold that endures only a second.
- **Discharge:** Totally loosen up your pelvic floor muscles as you return to your regular breathing musicality.
- **Rehash:** Perform 10 fast flicks straight, zeroing in on the speed and control of every constriction and delivery.

<u>**Supportive of Tips for beginners:**</u>

Center around Quality, Not Amount: Don't stress over doing a lot of speedy flicks immediately. Begin with a reasonable number (like 5-10) and spotlight on performing them with legitimate methods. Consistency is critical!

- **Try not to Pause Your Breathing:** Inhale regularly all through the activity. Pausing your breathing can strain your body and ruin the viability of the Kegel.
- **Loosen up Totally:** Recall, the unwinding stage is similarly just about as significant as the withdrawal. Completely delivering your pelvic floor muscles permits them to re-energize and prepare for the following fast flick.
- **Pay attention to Your Body:** In the event that you experience any distress, stop the activity and counsel a medical care proficient.

<u>**Feel the Distinction:**</u>

Fast Flick Kegels are an extraordinary method for building rate and control in your pelvic floor muscles. With predictable practice, you might encounter a few advantages, including:

<u>**Worked on urinary control**</u>

- Upgraded sexual endurance and execution
- More grounded center and better stance

Keep in mind, consistency is critical! Expect to do Fast Flick Kegels a couple of times each day, alongside your customary Kegel schedule, to see and feel the distinction.

Heel Slides

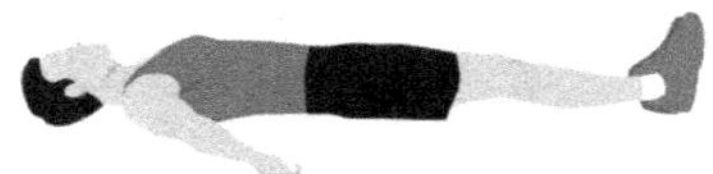

Heel slides are a phenomenal activity to integrate into your Kegel routine since they focus on your pelvic floor muscles in an exceptional manner. They consolidate the center commitment of a leg slide with the engaged compression of a Kegel, making them an incredible choice for fledglings who are as yet getting the hang of disengaging those muscles. This is the way to perform heel slides effortlessly:

What You'll Need:
- An agreeable mat or covered floor

Bit by bit Guide:

See as Your Base: Start by lying easily on your back with your knees bowed and feet level on the floor. Your knees ought to be hip-width separated, and your arms can rest serenely by your sides.

Draw in Your Center: Before you start the development, take a full breath and tenderly fix your center muscles. Envision pulling your midsection button inwards towards your spine. This makes a steady base for your body and safeguards your lower back during the activity.

Slide and Press: Presently comes the tomfoolery part! Center around getting your pelvic floor muscles, as though you're attempting to prevent yourself from passing pee halfway (however don't really attempt to stop pee). Here is the key: While holding this pelvic floor withdrawal, gradually slide one heel away from your body along the floor, keeping your leg straight. Try not to lift your heel totally off the ground, simply coast it easily.

Feel the Association: As you slide your heel, focus on the commitment to your pelvic floor. You ought to feel a slight fixing or lifting sensation profound inside. Keep in mind: There's actually no need to focus on the distance you slide your heel, however the nature of the withdrawal.

Slide Back and Rehash: When your heel arrives at its farthest agreeable point, gradually slide it back towards your body while keeping up with the pelvic floor crush. Envision bringing your heel back "home" to the beginning position.

Switch Sides and Rehash: Complete 8-12 redundancies with one leg, then tenderly lower that foot down and rehash the whole cycle with the other leg. You can go for the gold arrangements of this exercise per exercise meeting.

<u>Tips for Amateurs:</u>
1. **Try not to Overstretch:** Spotlight on a little, controlled slide instead of attempting to extend your leg excessively far. It means quite a bit to feel the commitment to your pelvic floor than to boost the distance your heel ventures.
2. **Inhale Simple:** Keep a consistent, loosened up breath all through the activity. Try not to pause your breathing while at the same time pressing your pelvic floor.
3. **Pay attention to Your Body:** On the off chance that you experience any aggravation or uneasiness, stop the activity and counsel your primary care physician prior to proceeding.
4. **Center around Quality, Not Amount:** Playing out a couple of redundancies with legitimate

structure than to do numerous reiterations with messy technique is better.

5. **Reward Tip:** As you become more OK with heel slides, you can add a little test by attempting them with a little towel set under the heel you're sliding. This makes some additional grinding and requires more center commitment to keep up with legitimate structure.

By integrating heel slides into your Kegel schedule, you'll be well en route to a more grounded pelvic floor, further developed center steadiness, and a freshly discovered appreciation for the smooth power inside you!

Happy Baby Pose

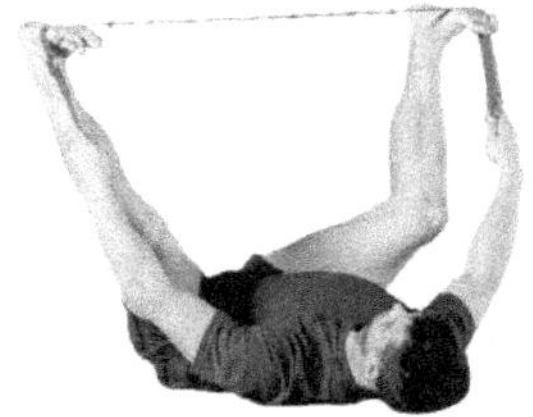

Have you at any point seen a child lying on their back, advantages in the air, getting a handle on their toes and shaking to and fro with joy? That is precisely the exact thing Blissful Child Posture (Ananda Balasana in Sanskrit) seems to be! This delicate and loosening up present is an ideal expansion to any yoga or novice's work-out daily practice, offering an astounding measure of advantage for your center and lower body.

This is the way to track down your inward blissful child, bit by bit:

1. See as Your Base:

Begin by lying serenely on your back on a yoga mat or a thick towel. Press your lower back level against the mat and extend your spine by tenderly pushing the crown of your head towards the floor. Take a couple of full breaths here, feeling your body subside into the posture.

2. Embrace Those Knees:

Bring your knees up towards your chest, keeping your shins opposite to the floor. Envision embracing your knees to your gut for a warm hug. Flex your feet, arching your foot towards the roof.

3. Reach and Spread:

Here comes the tomfoolery part! Arrive at your hands back and tenderly handle the external edges of your feet (or the inward bottoms assuming that is more agreeable). You can definitely relax on the off chance that you can't arrive at as far as possible from the beginning - utilize a yoga tie or towel circled around your curves for an additional help. Presently, tenderly spread your knees separated, meaning to bring them more extensive than your hips. Feel a decent stretch in your internal thighs? That is something to be thankful for!

4. Rock and Roll (Delicately):
This is where the enchantment occurs! With your hands holding your feet (or the tie), delicately rock from one side to another, imitating a cheerful child's energetic development. Envision influencing to and fro in a rocker. Inhale profoundly and center around the delicate shaking sensation. In the case of shaking feels awkward, basically hold the posture with your knees spread and inhale profoundly.

5. Track down Your Blissful Spot:
Remain in Cheerful Child Posture however long feels good, commonly something like 30 seconds to a moment for fledglings. Inhale profoundly and equally all through the posture, zeroing in on the delicate stretch and the impression of your center muscles tenderly captivating. At the point when you're prepared to emerge from the posture, gradually lower your knees back down to the mat, each in turn, and deliver your feet. Loosen up on your back for a couple of seconds, feeling the serenity and revival spreading through your body.

Reward Tip: For an additional test, have a go at shaking side-to-side while pressing your pelvic floor muscles (like doing a Kegel). This will add an additional layer of center commitment to the posture.

Keep in mind, Blissful Child Posture is tied in with seeing as a delicate stretch and feeling good. Try not to drive yourself into anything that feels agonizing. Stand by listening to your body, have some good times, and partake in the excursion to a more grounded, more loosened up you!

Lying Down

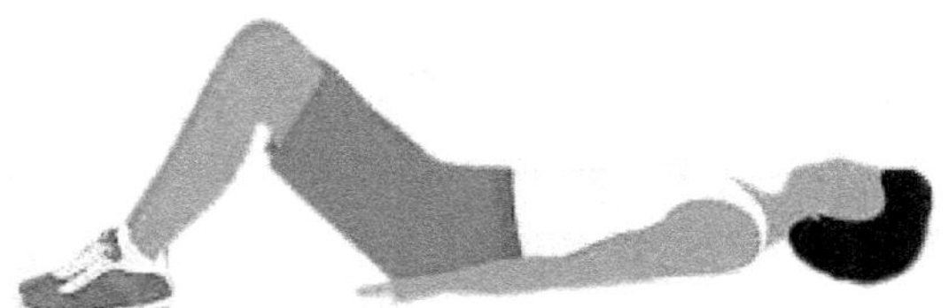

The resting position is a fabulous beginning stage for Kegel works out. particularly for fledglings. Here is a bit by bit manual for guarantee you're performing them accurately and receiving the rewards:

<u>**What You'll Need:**</u>

- An agreeable, calm space
- A yoga mat (discretionary)

<u>**Stage 1: Settle in**</u>

- Find a peaceful spot where you will not be interfered.
- Rests on your back with your knees bowed and feet level on the floor. You can put a yoga mat for added solace.
- Loosen up your shoulders and let your arms rest serenely at your sides.

<u>**Stage 2: Separate the Pelvic Floor Muscles**</u>

- Envision you're attempting to stop yourself halfway while you're utilizing the washroom. That is the essential Kegel compression! The muscles you're utilizing are your pelvic floor muscles, and they're similar to a lounger supporting your bladder, rectum, and regenerative organs.

<u>**Stage 3: The Crush and Delivery**</u>

- Presently, without grasping your rump or fixing your abs, tenderly crush your pelvic floor muscles upwards. Consider lifting them towards your spine.
- Hold the press for a count of 2-3 seconds. Center around the vibe of fixing those inner muscles.

- Loosen up your pelvic floor muscles totally. Envision delivering the crush and allowing all that to fall down normally. Build up to 2-3 seconds during this unwinding stage.

Stage 4: Rehash and Relax

- Rehash this succession of press hold-discharge for 10 redundancies. Make sure to inhale all through the activity. Breathe out as you contract and breathe in as you unwind.

Tips for Fledglings:

- Try not to strain or pause your breathing. Keep the activity delicate and controlled.
- It's alright on the off chance that you don't feel much from the start. With reliable practice, you'll turn out to be more mindful of your pelvic floor muscles and feel the compressions getting more grounded.
- Begin with more limited holds (2-3 seconds) and progressively increment them as you get more grounded (go for the gold 5-7 seconds).
- Center around better standards without compromise. Playing out a couple of reiterations with legitimate structure than numerous with erroneous technique is better.

Varieties for Added Challenge (When You're Agreeable):

Beats: Rather than holding the compression for a couple of moments, perform speedy heartbeats by crushing and delivering your pelvic floor muscles quickly. Go for the gold heartbeats.

Press and Lift: As you crush your pelvic floor muscles, attempt to lift your hips somewhat off the ground. Hold briefly, then lower your hips back down and unwind. Rehash this 5-10 times.

Keep in mind:

- Be patient and predictable with your Kegel works out! Go for the gold arrangements of 10 redundancies everyday, and step by step increment the recurrence and power as you get more grounded.

- Resting Kegels are a straightforward yet strong method for reinforcing your pelvic floor, further develop center steadiness, and experience a scope of medical advantages. In this way, unwind, inhale, and begin crushing your direction to a more grounded you!

Sitting

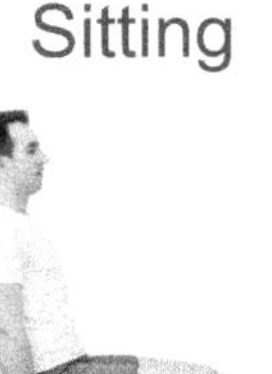
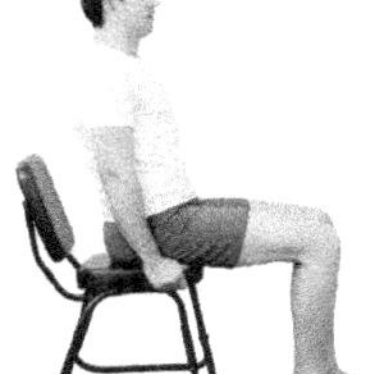

<u>1. Track down an Agreeable Seat:</u>

Pick a seat with a firm seat and great back help. Sit upstanding with your feet level on the floor, hip-width separated. Abstain from slumping - envision extending your spine and keeping your shoulders loose.

2. Connect with Your Center:

Take a full breath in, and as you breathe out, delicately fix your muscular strength. This will assist with balancing out your center and give an establishment to the Kegel workout.

3. Disconnect the Pelvic Floor Muscles:

Envision you're attempting to stop yourself halfway while you're utilizing the washroom. That is the fundamental sensation you're holding back nothing Kegel constriction. Try not to crush your hindquarters, thighs, or stomach - center around fixing the muscles inside your pelvis.

4. Agreement and Hold:

Whenever you've disconnected the inclination, tenderly press your pelvic floor muscles as though you're lifting them upwards. Hold this constriction for a count of 2-3 seconds.

5. Unwind and Rehash:

Gradually discharge the withdrawal and loosen up your pelvic floor muscles totally. Go for the gold redundancies of this arrangement.

Here are a few extra tips for fledglings doing Kegel practices in a sitting position:

- **Relax:** Make sure to inhale all through the activity. Breathe in as you unwind, and breathe out as you contract.
- **Center around Quality, Not Amount:** It means a lot to zero in on playing out a right compression than going for the gold number of redundancies. Begin with a couple of redundancies and bit by bit increment as you get more grounded.
- **Consistency is Vital:** Mean to do Kegel practices a couple of times each day, regardless of whether it's only a couple of sets. Consistency is a higher priority than long, rare meetings.
- **Pay attention to Your Body:** On the off chance that you experience any aggravation or uneasiness, stop the activity and counsel a specialist.

<u>**Reward Tip:**</u>

- Envision you're getting a little marble with your pelvic floor muscles. This perception can assist you with separating the right constriction.
- With just the right amount of training, you'll dominate the Kegel practice in a sitting position and be well headed to a more grounded pelvic floor!

Side Lying

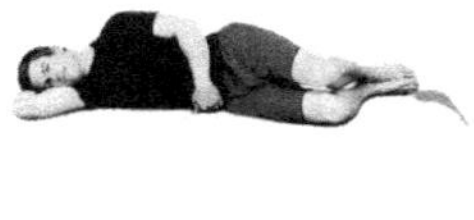

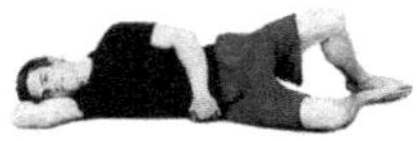

<u>**Why Side Lying?**</u>

The side-lying position is an incredible choice for fledglings since it offers a few advantages:

- **Unwinding:** Lying on your side can assist you with loosening up your body, making it more straightforward to disengage and zero in on your pelvic floor muscles.
- **Targets Explicit Muscles:** This position can assist with focusing on the slanted pelvic floor muscles, which add to by and large pelvic floor strength and backing.
- **Agreeable:** For certain people, side-lying could feel more good than lying level on their back, particularly those with back issues.

<u>**Step by step Guide:**</u>

1. **Find Your Usual range of familiarity:** Snatch a mat or delicate surface and rests on your side. You can pick either side - whichever feels more great for you. Twist your knees and stack them on top of one another.

2. **Unwind and Relax:** Take a couple of full breaths, zeroing in on relinquishing any strain in your body. Envision your spine protracting with each breathe in and relaxing with each breathe out.

3. **Secluding the Pelvic Floor:** Envision you're attempting to stop yourself halfway while utilizing the restroom. That is the fundamental Kegel constriction you'll zero in on. Fix your pelvic floor muscles as though you're doing exactly that, crushing inwards and upwards.

4. **Hold and Delivery:** Hold this constriction for a couple of moments (go for the gold seconds to begin). Make sure to inhale all through - breathe out as you contract and breathe in as you discharge.

5. **Rehash and Unwind:** Gradually discharge the constriction and loosen up your pelvic floor muscles totally. Rehash this course of contracting, holding, and delivering for 10-15 reiterations.

6. **Switch Sides:** Whenever you've finished your set on one side, delicately turn over and rehash the whole cycle on the opposite side.

<u>**Tips for Novices:**</u>

- Try not to tense your stomach, hindquarters, or thighs. Center exclusively around getting your pelvic floor muscles.

- It could take a couple of attempts to feel the right muscles lock in. Be patient and steady with your training.
- In the event that you experience any aggravation, stop the activity and counsel a medical services proficient.
- You can integrate side-lying Kegels into your day to day everyday practice - while staring at the television, perusing a book, or in any event, holding up in line.

Keep in mind: Consistency is vital! Plan to do Kegel practices in the side-lying position (or some other agreeable position) a couple of times each day. As you get more grounded, you can continuously build the span of the holds and the quantity of reiterations.

Hands and Knees

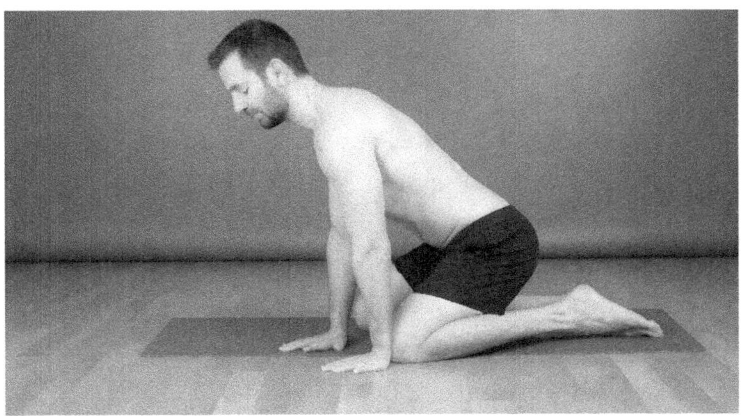

The hands and knees Kegel position is a fabulous choice for fledglings. It offers a delicate method for connecting with your center and pelvic floor muscles at the same time. Here is a bit by bit manual for dominating this position:

<u>What You'll Need:</u>
- An agreeable activity mat (discretionary)

<u>Steps:</u>
1. **Get down on the ground:** Begin by stooping on the floor with your hands straightforwardly under your shoulders.
2. **Track down an Impartial Spine:** Keep your back straight and abstain from curving your back or adjusting your shoulders. Imagine a straight line running from your head down your spine to your tailbone.

3. **Connect with Your Center:** Tenderly force your gut button in towards your spine, drawing in your center muscles. This will offer extra help for your lower back.

4. **The Kegel Press:** Presently comes the key part - the Kegel compression. Envision you're attempting to stop yourself halfway while utilizing the washroom. Press your pelvic floor muscles as though you're lifting them upwards. Hold this compression for a couple of moments (go for the gold seconds to begin).

5. **Relax:** Make sure to inhale all through the activity! Breathe in as you get ready for the compression, and breathe out leisurely as you discharge the crush.

6. **Unwind and Rehash:** Loosen up your pelvic floor muscles totally after the hold. Rehash stages 4-6 for 10-15 redundancies.

<u>**Tips for beginners:**</u>

- **Center around Quality, Not Amount:** from the beginning, center around playing out a legitimate Kegel compression with great structure as opposed to going for the gold number of reiterations.

- **Pay attention to Your Body:** Don't strain or pause your breathing. In the event that you feel any aggravation, stop the activity and counsel a medical care proficient.

- **Steadily Increment Power:** As you get more grounded, you can bit by bit expand the term of the hold and the quantity of reiterations.

<u>Advantages of Hands and Knees Kegels:</u>
- **Draws in Center:** This position normally actuates your center muscles, offering extra help for your spine and pelvis.
- **Further develops Coordination:** Organizing your breath with the Kegel compression can further develop your general body mindfulness.
- **Delicate on Novices:** The hands and knees position gives an agreeable and open method for rehearsing Kegels.

<u>Varieties for Cutting edge Clients:</u>
- **Leg Lifts:** While holding the Kegel withdrawal, gradually lift one leg off the ground, keeping your knee bowed. Hold briefly, then, at that point, bring down your leg and rehash with the opposite side.
- **Arm Lifts:** To challenge your center further, take a stab at taking one arm off the ground while keeping up with the Kegel constriction. Hold briefly, then bring down your arm and rehash with the opposite side.

Keep in mind, consistency is vital! Indeed, even a couple of sets of Kegels in the hands and knees position done consistently can have a major effect in reinforcing your center and pelvic floor.

Squatting

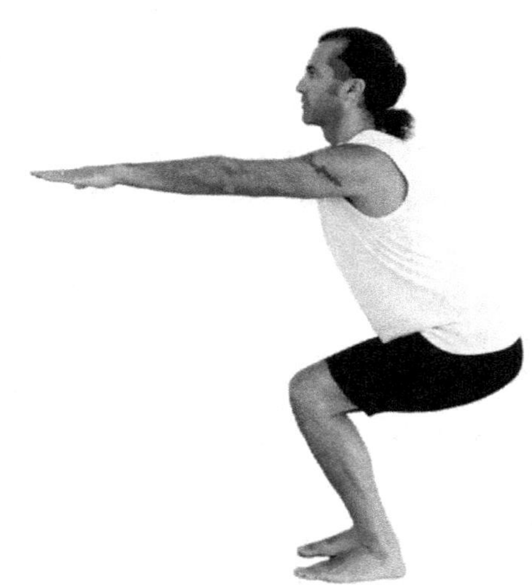

Squats could appear to be a basic activity, however trust me, they're a stalwart move that merits a spot in any gym routine daily practice. They're not just about etched legs (however that is a pleasant advantage!). Squats are the establishment for lower body strength, center initiation, and a sensation of strengthening that goes past the exercise center.

Here is step by step guide for dominating the ideal squat, particularly for novices:

<u>**Gear Up (let's start):**</u>

The excellence of squats is that you needn't bother with any extravagant hardware! You can do them anyplace, whenever, with simply your body weight. In any case, in the event that you feel more open to beginning with some help, you can involve a seat for a variety.

<u>**Prepare to Crouch!**</u>

- **Stand Tall:** Begin by remaining with your feet shoulder-width separated. Envision a straight line running from your lower legs through your hips and shoulders.
- **Connect with Your Center:** Envision pulling your gut button towards your spine to fix your center muscles. This will assist with settling your body during the squat.
- **Arrive at Back and Plunk Down:** Imagine you will plunk down in an undetectable seat! Pivot at your hips as though you're pushing your glutes back, and twist your knees simultaneously. Make sure you keep your back straight and your chest raised.

<u>**The Ideal Squat Profundity:**</u>

Here is a basic part for novices - how low would it be a good idea for you to go?

- **Hold back nothing:** an effective method for checking profundity is to ensure your thighs are generally lined up with the ground.

- **Knees Over Toes (Yet Not To an extreme!):**
  Your knees ought to follow over your toes, yet try
  not to allow them to buckle internally.

Propel Yourself Up (The Tomfoolery Part!):

Whenever you've arrived at your squat profundity, now
is the right time to rise! Connect with your glutes and
quads (the muscles on the front and back of your thighs)
to propel yourself back up to the beginning position.
Center around pushing through your heels for a strong
lift.

Rehash and Relax:

- Hold back nothing redundancies for a set. Make
  sure to inhale all through the development -
  breathe out as you lower yourself down, and
  breathe in as you propel yourself back up.

Favorable to Tips for Amateurs:

- **Keep a Straight Back:** Abstain from slouching
  your back during the squat. Keep a tall stance all
  through the development.

- **Look Forward:** Don't peer down at your feet!
  Keep your head in accordance with your spine
  and your look engaged forward.

- **Try not to Propel Yourself Excessively Hard:**
  Pay attention to your body. In the event that you
  feel any aggravation, stop the activity and
  counsel a specialist.

- **Dominating the Squat:** It's an Excursion, Not an
  Objective

Try not to get deterred in the event that your squats are flawed immediately. Practice gains ground! As you get more grounded, you can continuously expand the quantity of repetitions per set, or take a stab at holding loads while you squat (whenever you've dominated the bodyweight squat). Be that as it may, recall, legitimate structure is vital to keeping away from injury and augmenting adequacy.

All in all, would you say you are prepared to check squats out? Embrace the test, feel the consumer (positively!), and open the unimaginable advantages this straightforward activity brings to the table!

Single-Leg Bridge

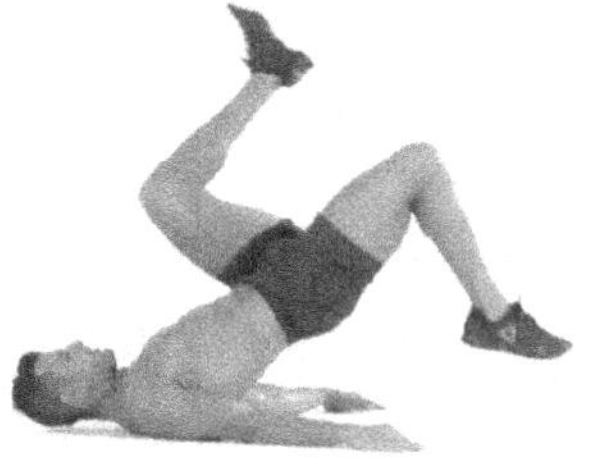

The Single-Leg bridge: Reinforcing Your Lower Body and Center

- The single-leg span is a fabulous activity that objectives your glutes, hamstrings, and center and further develops balance. It's an extraordinary movement from the customary scaffold exercise and adds a component of challenge. Here is a bit by bit manual for dominating the single-leg span, ideal for novices:

What You'll Need:

- An agreeable activity mat (discretionary)

Steps:

1. **Get Set Up:** Lie on your back with your knees bowed and feet level on the floor, hip-width separated. Your arms ought to rest easily by your sides with palms confronting.

2. **Lift One Leg:** Expand one leg straight up towards the roof, keeping your toes pointed. This will be the leg you're adjusting on.

3. **Connect with Your Center:** Support your center muscles as though you're going to be hit directly in the gut. This will assist with balancing out your spine and safeguard your lower back all through the activity.

4. **Press Up:** Push through the impact point of the established foot (the foot that is still on the ground) and lift your hips off the ground until your body frames a straight line from your shoulders to your drawn out knee. Envision crushing your glutes to start the vertical development.

5. **Hold and Press:** Stand firm on the extension footing briefly, zeroing in on crushing your glutes and keeping your center locked in. Ensure your hips stay level and try not to allow them to plunge towards the lifted leg.

6. **Lower Down:** Gradually lower your hips back down to the beginning situation in a controlled way. Try not to simply thud down!

7. **Rehash and Switch:** Complete the ideal number of redundancies (10-15 reps is a decent beginning stage) with a similar leg, then, at that point, bring down your leg and rehash the whole cycle with the other leg.

<u>Tips for Amateurs:</u>

- Center around Structure: Appropriate structure is essential to stay away from injury and augment viability. Focus on keeping your hips level, center connected with, and back straight all through the development.

- Begin with Bodyweight: Start by playing out the single-leg span with only your bodyweight. Whenever you've dominated the development with great structure, you can continuously add weight by holding a hand weight in each hand.

- Keep up with Control: Move gradually and purposely all through the activity. Keep away from jerky developments or racing through the redundancies.

- Pay attention to Your Body: In the event that you feel any aggravation, stop the activity and counsel a specialist or actual advisor.

<u>**Varieties for Added Challenge:**</u>

- **Single-Leg Extension with Heartbeat:** Whenever you've dominated the essential development, have a go at adding a heartbeat at the top. Arrive at the extension position, then perform little all over the place beats with your hips for a count of 2-3 preceding dropping down.
- **Single-Leg Scaffold with Arm Reach:** For an additional center test, expand one arm straight up towards the roof as you play out the single-leg span. Substitute arms with every reiteration.

<u>**The Single-Leg Extension: A Flexible Activity**</u>

The single-leg span is a basic yet strong activity that can be integrated into different exercise routine schedules. It's an extraordinary method for focusing on your lower body muscles, further developing center strength, and upgrade balance. Make sure to begin slowly, center around structure, and continuously increment the trouble as you get more grounded. With reliable practice, you'll be a solitary leg span genius quickly!

(For Advanced Individuals:) Kegel with Ball Squeeze

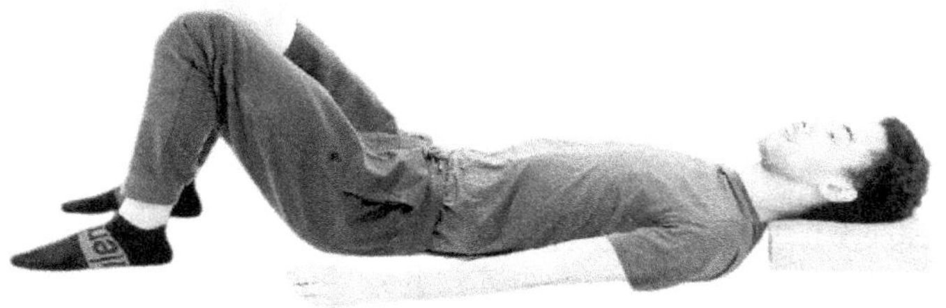

Kegel with Ball Press: Fortifying Your Pelvic Floor with an Additional Test

- The Kegel with Ball Press is a variety of the exemplary Kegel practice that adds a component of opposition, making it ideal for the individuals who need to take their pelvic floor preparing to a higher level. This is a bit by bit guide for fledglings:

<u>What You'll Need:</u>

A little activity ball, in a perfect world around the size of a tennis ball (yet pick an agreeable size for you)

<u>**Preparing:**</u>

- **Track down an Agreeable Position:** Pick a position where you can loosen up your body and spotlight on detaching your pelvic floor muscles. Lie on your back with your knees bowed and feet level on the floor is an incredible beginning stage.
- **Place the Ball:** Tenderly position the activity ball between your knees. You can change the situation relying upon your solace level - higher up for a more extraordinary press, or lower down for a gentler inclination.

<u>**Playing out the Activity:**</u>

1. **Connect with Your Center:** Prior to beginning the Kegel compression, delicately fix your center muscles as though drawing your gut button towards your spine. This gives strength and disconnects the pelvic floor muscles.

2. **Crush the Ball:** Envision you're attempting to press the ball between your knees. As you do this, contract your pelvic floor muscles as though you're halting yourself halfway when you utilize the washroom.

3. **Hold and Delivery:** Hold the constriction for a couple of moments (go for the gold seconds to begin) while keeping up with the press ready. Then, at that point, gradually loosen up both the pelvic floor muscles and your hold ready.

4. **Rehash and Relax:** Rehash this arrangement of crush, hold, and delivery for 10-15 reiterations. Make sure to inhale all through the activity - breathe out as you contract and breathe in as you unwind.

<u>**Tips for Fledglings:**</u>

- **Begin Slow:** Don't attempt to press the ball excessively hard or hold the compression for a really long time. Start with more limited holds and a delicate press, steadily expanding the power as your pelvic floor muscles get more grounded.

- **Pay attention to Your Body:** On the off chance that you experience any aggravation or distress, stop the activity and talk with a medical care proficient prior to proceeding.

- **Center around Strategy:** Appropriate structure is a higher priority than pressing the ball as hard as possible. Focus on getting your pelvic floor muscles, not simply pressing your thighs together.

- **Make it Fun:** Pick an activity ball in a variety you like or with a finished surface for added tactile excitement. You can likewise integrate the Kegel with Ball Get into your everyday daily practice - take a stab at doing it while sitting in front of the television or holding up in line.

<u>**Movement:**</u>

When you feel OK with the essential Kegel with Ball Crush, you can continuously expand the trouble:

- **Hold for Longer:** As your pelvic floor muscles reinforce, take a stab at holding the press and compression for a more drawn out span (as long as 10 seconds).
- **Quicker Presses:** Consolidate speedier, beating in the middle of between the more extended holds to target different muscle filaments.
- **Change Ball Position:** Examination with setting the ball sequentially between your knees to target various regions of your pelvic floor.

Keep in mind, consistency is critical! Expect to perform Kegel with Ball Press practices a couple of times each day, regardless of whether it's only a couple of establishes each point in time. With normal practice, you'll feel the distinction in your pelvic floor strength and generally prosperity.

walks with Kegels consistently can fundamentally fortify your pelvic floor muscles and further develop your general prosperity.

Chapter 3: Building a Sustainable Routine: Frequency, Consistency, and the Power of Progress

How Often Should You Practice Kegel Exercises?

Can we just be real, consistency can be a battle. We as a whole have those occasions when life confuses us, and that painstakingly arranged Kegel routine gets thrown to the side like the previous paper. However, listen to this, old buddy - consistency is the enchanted fixing that opens the genuine force of Kegels. It's the scaffold between "sincere goals" and "genuine outcomes."

Presently, I can actually read your mind: "How frequently is much of the time enough?" And trust me, when I initially began, I scoured the web for an enchanted number, a one-size-fits-all response. Be that as it may, here's the wonderful truth I've found: there isn't one. The "awesome" Kegel recurrence is however special as you may be.

Think about it like structure of a muscle. You couldn't anticipate seeing etched biceps after a solitary meeting at the exercise center, okay? The equivalent goes for your pelvic floor. Developing fortitude and perseverance takes time and commitment.

Be that as it may, here's the uplifting news: you don't have to devote hours to Kegels. Think little, feasible successes. Begin with a couple of sets of 10 redundancies per day. Perhaps three sets in the first part of the day, one more three preceding bed. The key is to find a musicality that fits flawlessly into your day to day everyday practice.

Here is a tip that made all the difference for me: Coordinate Kegels into your current propensities. Do a set while you clean your teeth, and one more while trusting that the pot will bubble. These little blasts accumulate over the long haul, and in a flash, Kegels become as normal as relaxing.

Keep in mind, consistency isn't about flawlessness. There will be days you miss a set, days when life gets insane. Try not to pound yourself! Simply get yourself, dust yourself off, and refocus. The significant thing is to continue to appear for your pelvic floor, little by little, step by step.

Furthermore, accept me, the outcomes are worth the effort. More grounded erections, further developed bladder control, and freshly discovered certainty - these are only a couple of the prizes that look for you in the way of predictable Kegel practice. Thus, embrace the excursion, track down your own mood, and watch your pelvic floor change into a force to be reckoned with of solidarity and sensation!

How Many Kegel Exercises Should a Man Do Per Day?

Ok, the million-dollar question, old buddy. At the point when I initially began with Kegels, I felt like I was suffocating in an ocean of clashing data. "Do 100 every day!" one site blast. "Begin with 5 and steadily increment!" one more forewarned. It was sufficient to blow your mind.

Here is reality I've realized: there's no enchanted number. Very much like any work-out daily practice, consistency is critical, however it's vital to pay attention to your body and find what turns out best for YOU.

Think about it like the structure of a muscle. You couldn't go to the exercise center and seat press the heaviest weight without skipping a beat, OK? You'd begin slowly, steadily increment the weight, and spotlight on legitimate structure. Kegels are the same.

This worked for me:

Begin little: Don't overpower yourself. Start with a reasonable number, similar to 5-10 Kegels per set, and spotlight on doing them accurately. Keep in mind, higher standards without compromise!

Pay attention to your body: As you get more grounded, you can slowly expand the quantity of repetitions per set. In any case, focus on any uneasiness. Slight touchiness is typical, yet torment is a warning.

- **Go for the gold:** better to do a couple of Kegels consistently than a hundred one day and afterward disregard them for seven days. Think about it like cleaning your teeth - an everyday propensity that prompts long haul benefits.
- **Here is a reward tip:** Separate your Kegels over the course of the day. Perhaps do a set while you're cleaning your teeth, one more while trusting that the pot will bubble, or even a couple of careful crushes while staring at the television. These little blasts add up and keep your pelvic floor connected over the course of the day.

At last, the quantity of Kegels you do is less significant than the responsibility you make to consistency. Track down a standard that feels quite a bit better for YOU, stay with it, and witness the astounding change in your pelvic floor wellbeing and generally prosperity. Trust me, your body (and perhaps your accomplice) will thank you for it!

Building a Sustainable Kegel Routine: Tips for Consistency

Can we just look at things objectively, folks. Consistency can be a genuine battle, particularly with regards to something as...unconventional as Kegels. Life tosses curves - work cutoff times, rec center meetings that leave you depleted, evenings spent spread on the sofa following a difficult day. In what would seem like no time, weeks have flown by, and your once-encouraging Kegel routine has turned into ancient history.

Be that as it may, here's what I've realized (the most difficult way possible, obviously): consistency is critical to opening the genuine force of Kegels. Think about it like structure muscle - those underlying presses could feel like a piece of cake, however with reliable exertion, you'll be flabbergasted at the strength and control you can create.

The issue is, how would we stay with it when life tosses its unavoidable wrenches? Indeed, old buddy, I've been there, and here are some fight tried tips that have assisted me with building a Kegel schedule that really sticks:

View as Your "Why": Can we just look at things objectively for a minute, inborn inspiration is a strong power. Dig profoundly and interface your Kegels to a greater objective. Is it about enduring longer in the room? Further developed bladder control? Perhaps it's just the fulfillment of assuming responsibility for your wellbeing. Whatever your explanation, record it on paper, and stick it on your washroom reflection - a steady sign of the "why" behind your endeavors.

Little Wins, Enormous Effect: Don't overpower yourself with ridiculous objectives. Begin little - a couple of sets of Kegels a day, regardless of whether it's only 5 presses each. Praise those little triumphs, and step by step increment the recurrence and span as you develop fortitude and certainty.

Make it Fun (Indeed, Truly!): Kegels don't need to be a task. Investigate the activity varieties I referenced before! Find what feels far better for you, what makes you grin. Perhaps it's imagining yourself driving a triumph march with those "Walk" Kegels, or perhaps it's the energetic delight of the "Cheerful Child Represent." A small amount of tomfoolery makes a huge difference in keeping you propelled.

Sneak them in the excellence of Kegels is their covertness. You can do them basically a place - at your work area while dealing with a report, trapped in rush hour gridlock, or even while sitting in front of the television (simply don't let your soul mate find you emulating that vehicle business excessively excitedly!).

Pal Up (or Application Up!): Responsibility is a useful asset. Enroll a companion (somebody tactful, obviously!) to go along with you on your Kegel venture. Challenge one another, share your encounters, and keep each other spurred. There are even accessible applications that can direct you through schedules and keep tabs on your development - a small amount of technical support can make an enormous difference.

Keep in mind, constructing a manageable Kegel routine is a long distance race, not a run. There will be days you miss, and days you feel deterred. However, don't pound yourself - simply pick yourself back up, dust yourself off, and refocus. The key is to be delicate with yourself, commend your advancement, and find what works for

YOU. With just enough imagination and these tips in your back pocket, you'll be well headed to opening the force of Kegels and receiving the rewards long into the future.

Chapter 4: Fueling Your Core: Optimizing Your Diet for Kegel Success

Understanding the Link Between Diet and Pelvic Floor Health

Can we just look at things objectively for a moment, folks. We as a whole know the significance of a sound eating regimen for our general prosperity. Yet, did you at any point stop to contemplate what you eat can mean for your, indeed, down-there wellbeing? It could sound bizarre, yet trust me, there's a strong association between your plate and the strength of your pelvic floor.

I'll concede, I used to move toward Kegels with a similar mentality. I moved toward my exercises - work it out, stretch myself to the edge, and stay optimistic. In any case, the outcomes were... disappointing. Then, I coincidentally found this captivating idea - the connection among diet and pelvic floor wellbeing. It was a distinct advantage.

Consider it along these lines. Your pelvic floor muscles resemble the ensemble guides of your lower areas. They control everything from urinary stream to sexual execution. Also, very much like any high-performing ensemble, they need the right fuel to sparkle really.

Here's where the sorcery of a solid eating regimen comes in. Envision throwing out the handled low quality food and supplanting it with a lively orchestra of natural products, vegetables, lean proteins, and entire grains. These stalwart fixings become the structure that blocks areas of strength for pelvic floor muscles.

Brace yourself for what I'm about to tell you, the thing that matters was amazing. Unexpectedly, my Kegel practices felt more effective. I saw a newly discovered control and endurance that basically wasn't there previously. It seemed like my body was at long last working with me, not against me.

Yet, it's not just about adding the great stuff. There are a few dietary offenders you want to keep under control. Consider them the shrieking violins that toss the entire symphony into confusion. Handled food sources, exorbitant sugar, and undesirable fats can prompt irritation, which can debilitate your pelvic floor muscles and leave them feeling drowsy.

Keep in mind, folks, assuming responsibility for your wellbeing is about something beyond heading out to the rec center. It's tied in with powering your body from the back to front. By embracing an eating routine wealthy in the right supplements, you're not simply giving your body the devices it requires to flourish, you're giving your pelvic floor muscles the fuel they hunger for to perform at their pinnacle. Thus, ditch the garbage, embrace the great stuff, and watch your Kegel venture change into an orchestra of progress!

Foods to Embrace for a Stronger Core

Can we just look at things objectively for a minute, folks. With regards to reinforcing our center, our brains frequently leap to perpetual crunches and rec center meetings. In any case, consider the possibility that I let you know there was a distinct advantage going unnoticed without really having to try, a flavorful method for building an unshakable center from the back to front. Truth be told, I'm discussing food - the fuel that controls our bodies and, in all honesty, assumes a vital part in the soundness of our pelvic floor.

For quite a while, I moved toward food with a "more will be more" mindset. The greater the burger, the better the exercise, isn't that so? Wrong. I before long understood that the oily cheap food I was scooping down wasn't helping my center. Truth be told, it was leaving me slow, swelled, and in all honesty, somewhat crushed.

However at that point, I found the wizardry of supplement rich food varieties. It wasn't necessary to focus on hardship, it was tied in with embracing a better approach for eating, a way that sustained my body and energized my exercises (and Kegels!). I realized this:

The Rainbow Mob: Recall those youth days spent picking the most brilliant, most vivid leafy foods? Ends up, there's a justification behind that wistfulness. These energetic forces to be reckoned with are loaded with fundamental nutrients, minerals, and cell reinforcements that keep us solid as well as add to major areas of strength for a story. Consider them minuscule champions battling irritation and supporting our center muscles from the back to front. So whenever you're at the supermarket, set your internal identity free and embrace the rainbow!

Lean and Mean Protein Power: Imagine yourself after an exceptional exercise, areas of strength for feeling invigorated. That is the sort of feeling protein gives.

Lean sources like chicken, fish, and beans are the structure blocks of muscle, and prepare to have your mind blown. Our pelvic floor muscles are no special case. Remembering these protein forces to be reckoned with for your eating regimen assists with post-exercise recuperation as well as supports the development and upkeep of solid pelvic floor muscles.

Entire Grain Miracles: Trench the handled white bread and refined carbs, my companions. Entire grains are the superheroes of the sugar world. Loaded with fiber, they keep you feeling full and stimulated over the course of the day. However, more critically, they assist with directing your stomach related framework, which is a vital part of keeping a solid pelvic floor. Consider them the quiet gatekeepers of your center, keeping everything working without a hitch.

Solid Fat Awesome: Fat. The actual word can send shudders down certain spines. However, here's reality: solid fats are fundamental for our general wellbeing, and that incorporates our pelvic floor. Food sources like avocados, nuts, and greasy fish are stacked with great for-you fats that help chemical equilibrium and might in fact further develop blood stream - both critical variables for a sound pelvic floor. Thus, embrace the great fats, and make it a point to add some avocado to your toast or partake in a modest bunch of almonds for a wonderful bite.

Keep in mind, folks, this isn't about limitation, about embracing heavenly food sources that work for yourself as well as your center. Consider it an interesting culinary experience, an opportunity to investigate new flavors and surfaces while giving your body the fuel it requirements to flourish. Thus, ditch the oily cheap food, get a rainbow of products of the soil, and leave on a tasty excursion to a more grounded, better you!

Fruits and Vegetables: Packed with Essential Nutrients

Can we just be real, foods grown from the ground haven't forever been the rockstars of our eating regimens. We've all been there - attracted to the alarm tune of sweet treats and oily pleasures. However, here's reality I've scholarly: foods grown from the ground aren't some exhausting discipline; they're nature's ensemble of flavor and imperativeness, ready to be investigated!

Recollect a period you chomped into an entirely ready strawberry - the blast of pleasantness on your tongue, the lively red juice staining your fingers. Or on the other hand perhaps it was the fantastic smash of a new carrot, its gritty flavor an unforeseen pleasure. These are the minutes that remind us why products of the soil are something beyond food; they're an encounter that stirs our faculties and feeds our spirits.

Be that as it may, the enchantment goes far past taste. These beautiful marvels are nature's forces to be reckoned with, loaded with fundamental supplements that keep our bodies murmuring. Recall that drowsy inclination after an oily feast? Products of the soil, then again, are overflowing with nutrients, minerals, and cell reinforcements that give us supported energy and a sound gleam.

This is how things have been: envision your body as a brilliant ensemble. Products of the soil are the instruments, every one assuming a crucial part in making wonderful music. The fresh mash of an apple may be the percussion, keeping the mood consistent. The energetic orange of yam could be the metal segment, adding an eruption of energy. Also, mixed greens? Consider them the quieting strings, giving fundamental agreement.

In this way, the following time you go after a tidbit, pause for a minute to investigate the rainbow on your plate. Let the succulent pleasantness of a mango entice your taste buds. Enjoy the reviving smash of a cucumber cut. Keep in mind, you're not simply supporting your body; you're taking care of your imperativeness, your energy, and your general prosperity. Trust me, when you treat leafy foods as the rockstars they genuinely are, your body will thank you for the delightful ensemble you're making inside.

<u>Lean Protein Sources: Building Blocks for Muscle Strength</u>

Can we just look at things objectively, it isn't not difficult to assemble muscle. It takes commitment, sweat, and perhaps a couple of tears (particularly after leg day, isn't that so?). In any case, there's one thing that isolates those end of the week fighters from the ladies and gentlemen who genuinely shape their fantasy physical make-ups - protein. It's the enchanted fixing, the foundation, the fuel that controls your muscle-building motor.

Presently, before you coat over at the prospect of another dry nourishment guide, listen to me. Since protein isn't just about tasteless chicken bosoms and protein shakes (despite the fact that, hello, there's a spot for those as well). It's about a culinary experience, an opportunity to investigate delightful, healthy food sources that sustain your body as well as light your taste buds.

Recall that inclination after an especially exhausting exercise? Legs consuming, lungs shouting, yet where it counts, a feeling of achievement that washes over you like a wave? That is the inclination protein assists you with pursuing. The information you're investing the effort, taking care of your body the right instruments, and gradually, without a doubt, chiseling the build you merit.

In any case, protein isn't just about style (however can we just look at things objectively, looking great feels pretty darn great). It's tied in with developing fortitude, flexibility, and certainty that transmits from the back to front. It's tied in with handling that additional rep, stretching your boundaries, and feeling the crude power flooding through your body. It's tied in with realizing you can vanquish any test life tosses your direction, both in the rec center and then some.

Presently, where do we find these supernatural protein sources? Lock in, on the grounds that we're going to leave on a flavor-stuffed venture!

Chicken: The OG, However Make it Intriguing

We should be genuine, chicken gets unfavorable criticism for being exhausting. In any case, prepare to be blown away. It's a lean protein force to be reckoned with which is as it should be! Try to discard the tasteless everyday practice and get inventive. Marinate your chicken in an ensemble of flavors, barbecue it to delicious flawlessness, and match it with broiled vegetables for a total feast that overflows with flavor. Or on the other hand, what about preparing a pan fried food with bright veggies and a light sauce? Chicken is your fresh start - paint it with your culinary inventiveness!

Fish: Jump into a Universe of Omega-3 Goodness

Calling all fish darlings! Salmon, fish, and cod - these aren't simply scrumptious choices, they're loaded with omega-3 unsaturated fats, fundamental for by and large wellbeing and muscle recuperation. Picture an impeccably burned salmon steak, shimmering with lemon margarine, or a light and flaky fish salad stacked with new dill. Fish offers a protein punch with a heart-solid reward - a shared benefit for your muscles and your prosperity.

Eggs: A Morning meal (and Then some) Champion

Eggs aren't only for breakfast any longer! These flexible protein bombs are a phenomenal wellspring of complete protein, meaning they contain every one of the fundamental amino acids your body needs. Scramble them with veggies for a morning shot in the arm, or prepare a protein omelet for a post-exercise refuel. Eggs are reasonable, helpful, and quite delectable - a genuine boss in any competitor's kitchen.

Vegetables: The Plant-Based Force to be reckoned with

Calling all veggie lovers and vegetarians! Tune in up, on the grounds that vegetables are your protein BFFs. Beans, lentils, chickpeas - these folks are overflowing with protein, fiber, and an abundance of other fundamental supplements. Prepare a good lentil soup to warm you up on a chilly day, or prepare chickpeas into a lively serving of mixed greens for a protein-stuffed lunch. Vegetables demonstrate that plant-based protein can be similarly essentially as delectable and fulfilling as its creature partners.

Greek Yogurt: A Velvety Protein Fix

Think yogurt is only for dessert? Reconsider! Greek yogurt, with its out of this world protein content and lower sugar levels contrasted with normal yogurt, makes for a fabulous post-exercise nibble or a light breakfast choice. Top it with berries, granola, or a sprinkle of honey for a fantastic and protein-rich treat.

Tofu and tempeh frequently get negative criticism, however they can be culinary chameleons when arranged accurately. Marinate your tofu in your #1 sauce, then, at that point, sear it to fresh flawlessness. Or on the other hand, disintegrate tempeh and add it to a pan fried food for a substantial surface. These soy-based choices are shockingly flexible and an extraordinary wellspring of plant-based protein.

This is only a sample of the staggering universe of lean protein sources ready to be investigated. Keep in mind, building muscle isn't about hardship; it's tied in with energizing your body with heavenly, healthy food varieties that sustain your muscles and fulfill your taste buds. Thus, ditch

Whole Grains: Providing Sustained Energy

At any point felt that recognizable evening droop? You know the one - the one where your eyelids get weighty, your mind feels like mush, and that tasty morning latte appears to be ancient history? No doubt, me as well. For quite a long time, I was a captive to the sugar crash cycle. Go after a sweet breakfast, experience a concise explosion of energy, and afterward fall into an efficiency void. It was only after I found the enchantment of entire grains that my relationship with energy totally changed.

You will scarcely believe, it wasn't love at first nibble. I experienced childhood with a consistent eating regimen of white bread, sweet oats, and handled snacks. Entire grains appeared to be some sort of wellbeing food craze, a universe of cardboard-tasting earthy colored rice and dull cereal. Yet, distress (and an earnest longing to jettison the midday droop) at last pushed me to check them out. What's more, you will scarcely believe it was a disclosure.

The principal thing I saw was the distinction in how my body utilized the energy. Gone were the anxious ups and pounding downs of the sugar rollercoaster. All things considered, entire grains gave a consistent, supported progression of energy that endured over the course of the morning. I could at long last zero in on undertakings, power through exercises, and feel truly present over the course of the day. It resembled a light switch that had been flipped inside me.

Be that as it may, the advantages went far past keeping away from the feared crash. Stop and think for a minute, entire grains are loaded with mind blowing supplements - fiber, nutrients, minerals, everything. Also, prepare to be blown away. These supplements don't simply fuel your body, they feed it. I began feeling lighter, and more empowered, and, surprisingly, my mind-set appeared to get to the next level. Perhaps it was the newly discovered certainty of overcoming the midday droop, or perhaps it was the wizardry of entire grain goodness working its miracles.

Presently, I'm not saying you need to turn into an entire grain perfectionist short-term. It all makes sense to me, some of the time a fleecy white bagel simply sounds darn engaging. In any case, here's the excellence, all things considered, - integrating entire grains into your eating regimen doesn't need to be a win big or bust recommendation. Begin little! Trade out your white bread for entire wheat toast. Sneak some quinoa into your next salad. Indeed, even a sprinkle of entire grain oats on your morning yogurt can have an effect. The key is to track down ways of incorporating them into your current everyday practice, making little moves that lead to large outcomes.

What's more, trust me, the outcomes are worth the effort. Past the supported energy and by and large prosperity, there's a feeling of strengthening that accompanies energizing your body with great, healthy food. You're not simply snatching a handy solution, you're putting resources into yourself, in your wellbeing, and in your capacity to make every second count.

Listen to this, life is an excursion, and it's quite a lot more charming when you have the energy to encounter it really. Envision handling that difficult climb with enduring endurance. Picture enduring a work show with careful attention. Imagine partaking in an exciting day with your family without surrendering to fatigue. That is the force of entire grains, my companions. They're not simply food, they're an accomplice in making a lively, vigorous life.

Thus, the following time you go after a tidbit or plan your dinners, think about trying entire grains out. You may very well find a relationship that changes your relationship with energy, engages your body, and opens a universe of potential outcomes you never knew existed. Furthermore, hello, if my excursion from sugar-crash casualty to entire grain lover can rouse you, then, at that point, that makes it all the really fulfilling. How about we ditch the midday droop together and embrace the force of supported energy with each tasty chomp!

Healthy Fats: Supporting Hormone Balance

Can we just look at things objectively, with regards to wellbeing exhortation, fat frequently gets unfavorable criticism. We've been barraged with messages about "low-fat" everything, leaving us with a twisted perspective on these fundamental supplements. In any case, here's reality I've found on my own wellbeing process: sound fats are not the adversary - they're the unaccounted for part in the hormonal congruency puzzle.

Everything began with a baffling exciting ride. My feelings were out of control, my energy levels plunged like a defective rollercoaster, and overlooked a decent night's rest - it seemed like ancient history. I accused pressure, obviously, however something more profound felt off. I dove into the universe of ladies' wellbeing, exploring all that from rest cleanliness to stretch administration. While these were useful bits of the riddle, a solitary article about the connection between sound fats and chemical equilibrium provoked my interest.

Captivated, I began digging further. What I found was a disclosure. Our bodies depend on solid fats to produce fundamental chemicals like estrogen, progesterone, and testosterone. These chemicals are the ensemble guides of our prosperity, affecting everything from mind-set guidelines to digestion and even drive. At the point when our eating regimen needs solid fats, this hormonal ensemble goes off-key.

However, the excursion wasn't about aimlessly adding fat to all that I ate. It was tied in with settling on cognizant decisions, trading out the awful immersed and trans fats for the heroes - the sound fats. Recollect those oily takeout feasts I believed were "treats"? They were supplanted with lively avocado toast (indeed, the publicity is genuine!), rich almond spread on entire wheat wafers, and salmon so flavorful it seemed like a festival.

The change was steady yet unquestionable. My emotional episodes relaxed, supplanted by a recently discovered feeling of close to home steadiness. My energy levels began to climb, and those subtle tranquil evenings at last returned. It wasn't just about feeling "better" - it was tied in with feeling such as myself once more, the lively, enthusiastic lady I realized I could be.

However, the enchantment of solid fats goes past private experience. Here is the science that backs it up:

1. **Strong MCTs:** Medium-chain fatty substances, found in coconut oil and grass-took care of margarine, are promptly consumed by the body and utilized for energy. This means a more steady temperament and supported energy levels, keeping those midday droops under control.

2. **Omega-3 Power:** Greasy fish like salmon, sardines, and mackerel are overflowing with omega-3 unsaturated fats, fundamental for solid mind capability. They likewise assume a part in directing irritation, which can disturb hormonal equilibrium.

3. **The Monounsaturated Wonders:** Avocados, olive oil, and nuts are wealthy in monounsaturated fats, known to further develop insulin responsiveness and backing solid glucose levels. Stable glucose implies less hormonal changes, prompting a more quiet, more adjusted you.

Presently, don't misunderstand me. This excursion wasn't consistently daylight and rainbows. There were snapshots of disarray (who knew exploring the fat path at the supermarket could so overpower?). There were even days when the alarm tone of an oily burger felt enticing. However, here's the clear-cut advantage I found: information is power. The more I found out about the positive effect of sound fats, the simpler it became to go with cognizant decisions.

Keep in mind, there's no need to focus on flawlessness. It's about progress. Each sound fat you integrate into your eating routine is a stage towards hormonal congruity. Here are a few hints to kick you off:

1. **Begin Little:** Don't redesign your whole eating regimen short-term. Start by adding a sprinkle of nuts to your cereal, trading your typical cooking oil for olive oil, or partaking in a cut of avocado toast for breakfast.

2. **Embrace Trial and error:** Solid fats arrive in a delightful assortment! Investigate various sorts of fish, nuts, and seeds to find what you appreciate most. Broiling your own nuts adds a superb crunch and permits you to control the salt substance.

3. **Get to know Sound Fats:** Consider them partners as you continue looking for hormonal equilibrium. They're not the adversary prowling on your plate - they're the clear-cut advantage ready to be released!

The excursion to hormonal congruity is an individual one. Be that as it may, by embracing solid fats, you're giving your body the structure blocks it necessitates to make an orchestra of prosperity. So ditch the apprehension, investigate the delectable universe of solid fats, and watch your body and brain sing fitting together. You have the right to feel astonishing and trust me, these overlooked yet truly great individuals can be your unmistakable advantage to accomplishing only that.

Chapter 5: Foods to Minimize: Keeping Your Core Clean

Processed Foods and Added Sugars: The Inflammatory Culprits

Can we just look at things objectively - life is occupied. Between work cutoff times, family responsibilities, and the ceaseless social spin, in some cases a good dinner feels like a far off dream. We go after the convenient solutions, the microwave meals, and the sweet tidbits that guarantee comfort in a brilliantly shaded bundle. In any case, here's reality: I've learned the most difficult way possible: those handled enticements frequently accompany a secret expense - a stewing fire of irritation that can unleash devastation on our bodies and brains.

For a really long time, I was a perfect example for the handled food trap. Cheap food snacks were my standard, sweet beverages energized my evenings, and frozen meals made all the difference (or so I thought) on occupied evenings. It was only after a tireless flood of weariness, unexplained throbs, and a general sensation of "blah" got comfortable that I at last halted to scrutinize my decisions. Was everything in my mind? Or on the other hand was there something more vile influencing everything?

An excursion to the specialist validated my intuitions: constant second rate irritation. Evidently, my relationship with handled treats was unobtrusively taking up arms inside me. The specialist barraged me with clinical language, yet the message was clear: my body was continually fully on guard, combating the fiery reaction set off by the handled food varieties I was eating.

It was a reminder, a boisterous and evident one. In any case, where do you try to start when your whole eating regimen has been based on accommodation? Truly, I felt overpowered. However at that point, a flash of assurance lit inside me. I won't allow handled food varieties to direct my wellbeing any longer. I planned to retaliate, one delectable, entire food at a time.

My process was difficult. The primary supermarket trip was a stunner. Out of nowhere, racks spilling over with splendidly shaded bundles changed into a minefield of stowed away sugars, unfortunate fats, and a clothing rundown of unpronounceable fixings. Be that as it may, with each name I examined, I felt a developing feeling of strengthening. Information turned into my weapon, and the more I found out about the fiery impacts of handled food varieties, the more resolved I became to break free.

In all actuality, handled food varieties are experts of camouflage. They're stacked with added sugars that take on the appearance of honest flavors, undesirable fats that hide underneath captivating surfaces, and an ensemble of counterfeit fixings that confound our bodies. These handled lowlifes disturb our stomach wellbeing, debilitate our safe framework, and make a constant fiery express that can appear in a large number of ways - weariness, throbs, mind haze, and even emotional episodes.

Yet, here's the uplifting news: our bodies are inconceivably versatile. When I began supplanting handled food varieties with entire, pure fixings, the change was momentous. The weariness lifted, the hurts died down, and a newly discovered clearness supplanted the cerebrum mist. It wasn't just about feeling quite a bit improved, however that was positively a much needed development. It was tied in with rediscovering a feeling of imperativeness and get-up-and-go that had been covered underneath the handled food fog.

It wasn't all daylight and rainbows, obviously. There were desires, and snapshots of shortcoming when the alarm tune of a helpful frozen supper took steps to pull me back in. In any case, with each longing for vanquished, my purpose developed further. I found a totally different universe of flavors through new foods grown from the ground, the delightful wealth of entire grains, and the protein influence of lean meats and vegetables. Cooking turned into an experience, not a task, and the most common way of feeding my body with genuine food changed into a wonderful demonstration of self esteem.

This isn't a prevailing fashion diet or a handy solution. It's a promise to a better, more joyful you. It's tied in with figuring out the force of food and deciding to fuel your body with fixings that sustain it, not arouse it. It's tied in with dumping the handled food trap and embracing a universe of lively flavors, recently discovered energy, and a feeling of prosperity that transmits from the back to front.

Thus, old buddy, in the event that you're feeling the impacts of constant poor quality aggravation assuming that the handled food trap makes them feel drowsy and in a bad way, I ask you to go along with me on this excursion. It will not be simple, yet trust me, it's worth the effort. How about we trade the handled garbage for genuine food, find the scrumptious capability of nature's abundance, and recover the energetic wellbeing we as a whole merit. Together, we should cut back the volume on irritation and light an orchestra of prosperity inside ourselves.

Excessive Saturated and Trans Fats: Hindering Blood Flow

Can we just be real, food is a wellspring of solace, festivity, and unadulterated happiness. It sustains our bodies, energizes our days, and unites us with friends and family. Yet, in some cases, the things we love the most can hold onto stowed away risks. That is the narrative of soaked and trans fats - a story I know quite well.

For quite a long time, I carried on with a day to day existence energized by comfort. Inexpensive food snacks, late-night fries, and those very enticing cakes - they were my go-to mates. Certainly, I realized they weren't the best decisions, yet the taste was obviously fulfilling. It was only after I began seeing an adjustment of myself that I understood the quiet conflict these fats were pursuing on my body.

The primary sign was laziness. That once-springy move toward my morning walk turned into a drag. Steps that I used to overcome effortlessly now amazed me. My exercises, when a wellspring of energy and achievement, felt like a task. It resembled a cover that had been drawn over my essentialness, denying me of the zing I once had.

Concerned, I dug further. Vast long periods of examination on the web, specialist visits, and conferences with nutritionists laid out an unmistakable picture: the guilty party - my unfortunate relationship with immersed and trans fats. They were like minuscule, treacherous beasts, obstructing my courses and preventing the smooth progression of blood all through my body. This absence of an appropriate blood stream implied less oxygen arrived at my muscles, leaving them drained and drowsy.

The disclosure was a punch to the stomach. I was right here, unconsciously undermining my own wellbeing with each chomp. Be that as it may, rather than floundering in self indulgence, I chose to retaliate. It was difficult. There were desires, snapshots of shortcoming, and days when that oily burger seemed like the least demanding choice. Yet, with each step, with each better decision, I began to feel a shift.

The drowsiness gradually started to blur. My morning strolls became brisker, the steps less overwhelming. That flash of energy began to return, and with it, a restored feeling of good faith. It wasn't just about actual prosperity; it was tied in with recovering my vitality.

This excursion has shown me a significant illustration: the food we pick significantly affects how we feel, both genuinely and inwardly. Immersed and trans fats could entice our taste buds, however the drawn out results can take our essence, denying us of the encounters that genuinely advance our lives.

Thus, we should discuss these secret adversaries. Immersed fats, tracked down in greasy meats, spread, and some dairy items, can develop in our conduits, prompting a condition called atherosclerosis. This limiting of the courses confines blood stream, making it harder for oxygen and supplements to arrive at our organs and tissues. Trans fats, the despicable twins made through a cycle called hydrogenation, are surprisingly more terrible. They raise terrible cholesterol (LDL) yet in addition lower great cholesterol (HDL), further steering the results towards coronary illness.

Be that as it may, dread not, my companions! This isn't a story without trust. The uplifting news is, we have the ability to modify the story. By going with cognizant decisions about what we eat, we can engage ourselves to assume back command over our wellbeing and recover our essentialness. How it's done:

1. **Turn into a Name Investigator:** Figure out how to peruse food marks like a master. Search for words like "immersed fat" and "trans fat." Assuming the numbers are high, set that thing back on the rack.

2. **Embrace the Force of Plants:** Natural products, vegetables, and entire grains are loaded with supplements and sound fats. Fill your plate with these dynamic tones and rediscover the delight of genuine food.

3. **Solid Fats are Your Companions:** Don't fear all fats! Unsaturated fats, similar to those tracked down in olive oil, avocados, and nuts, are fundamental for good wellbeing. They assist with bringing down terrible cholesterol and advance in general prosperity.

4. **Cook More at Home:** This gives you unlimited authority over the fixings that go into your dinners. Try different things with solid recipes, find new flavors and make cooking a pleasant encounter.

Keep in mind, this isn't about hardship; it's about strengthening. About picking food sources sustain your body and fuel your soul. It's tied in with feeling the spring back in your step, the energy to pursue your fantasies, and the essentialness to appreciate each experience life offers. Thus, ditch the soaked and trans fats, embrace a better way of life, and recover the dynamic you have been standing by to break free. Your whole body, your brain, and your soul will thank you for it.

Excessive Caffeine and Alcohol: Potential Disruptors

Can we just look at things objectively for a moment, life can be a tenacious dance among efficiency and loosening up. We shuffle work cutoff times, family responsibilities, and that consistently present longing for a tad "personal time." In this hurricane, it's not difficult to go after the two most normal colleagues - the morning cup of joe and the night glass of wine. In any case, consider the possibility that I let you know this apparently innocuous pair may be playing a slippery game in the background, unleashing ruin on your prosperity.

My story started like numerous others. The relentless fragrance of newly blended espresso was my reminder, a shock of energy to overcome the day. It powered my desire and obscured the lines among exhaustion and concentration. However, incidentally, that dependable cup transformed into a support. Three, four, or even five cups turned into the standard, every one promising an explosion of energy that never fully endured. A bad case of nerves turned into a dependable friend, my stomach a beating wreck. Rest, when an ecstatic departure, transformed into a war zone. Thrashing around, my psyche dashed with the day's concerns, energized by the waiting impacts of caffeine.

Depletion turned into my unwanted visitor. The very thing I looked for - efficiency - was falling through my grip. My disappointment mounted. I felt like a hamster on a wheel, unendingly running however never arriving at the end goal. It was a reminder, a severe one conveyed by the very substance I depended on.

Then, at that point, came the nights. Wine, with its commitment of unwinding, turned into my compensation following a difficult day. A glass, perhaps two, appeared to be sufficiently innocuous. It dissolved away the pressure, for some time. In any case, the following morning, the haze returned, heavier and more persevering. My once-sharp center dwindled, supplanted by a dull throb in my mind and a general feeling of languor. My temperament, when raised by the impermanent break, dove, leaving me peevish and touchy.

It was an endless loop. I desired the caffeine to battle the drowsiness welcomed on by the liquor, and the liquor to dull the edge of the caffeine butterflies. I was trapped in a self-caused back-and-forth, my body the reluctant milestone.

Be that as it may, stop and think for a minute, dear peruser, this doesn't need to be your story. There's a method for breaking liberated from this troublesome couple. It was difficult, however I tracked down a way towards a better, more adjusted me. I realized this:

The Tricky Appeal of Caffeine:

We as a whole realize caffeine gives us an impermanent jolt of energy. In any case, what we frequently neglect is that it's an energizer, basically fooling our bodies into believing they're more ready than they really are. This acquired energy includes some significant downfalls. After some time, caffeine can disturb our normal rest wake cycle, prompting a sleeping disorder, tension, and, surprisingly, stomach related issues. Recollect that cup that vowed to keep you sharp? It very well may be the very thing thwarting your concentration and lucidity.

Liquor: The Misleading Companion:

That first impression of unwinding after a glass of wine? It's underhanded. Liquor could quiet you into a misguided feeling of quiet, however it disturbs your rest cycle in an unobtrusive yet huge manner. It smothers REM rest, the stage fundamental for memory solidification and profound guideline. No big surprise you awaken feeling hazy and bad tempered - your cerebrum just hasn't gotten the opportunity to re-energize appropriately.

Breaking Free: An Excursion of Self-Revelation

It was difficult, yet I progressively weaned myself off the over the top caffeine and liquor reliance. It implied dealing with my weariness directly, focusing on rest cleanliness, and creating better survival techniques for stress.

This aided me:

- **Hydration is Critical:** I supplanted those additional cups of espresso with water. Remaining hydrated assists your body with working ideally as well as battles the getting dried out impacts of caffeine. In all honesty, water can really give you a characteristic jolt of energy.
- **Pay attention to Your Body's Mood:** Rather than depending on caffeine to ride out the midday

droop, I began focusing on my body's regular energy plunges. A short walk or some careful stretching did ponder for resuscitating my concentration.

Tracking down Quieting Ceremonies: Rather than going after a glass of wine, I investigated alternate ways of loosening up. Washing up, perusing a book, or rehearsing profound breathing activities turned into my go-to pressure relievers. These exercises quieted my brain as well as permitted me to nod off normally.

The Awards of Equilibrium

The change, while slow, was amazing. My rest improved, and with it, my concentration and energy levels took off. The steady nerves and evening crashes turned into ancient history. My temperament balanced out, and my general prosperity

Chapter 6: Beyond the Basics: Exploring Advanced Techniques for Experienced Men

Fast Kegels vs. Slow Kegels: Tailoring Your Routine for Specific Goals

<u>Fast Kegels: Enhancing Control and Stamina</u>

Can we just look at things objectively for a minute, folks. We as a whole need to be the lords of endurance in the room. Flabbergasting our accomplices and ourselves feeling like heroes is irrefutably engaging. In any case, accomplishing that degree of control and perseverance can feel like a far off dream, particularly as we age or face specific wellbeing challenges.

That is where the universe of Kegels enters the image. We've all heard the murmurs, the modest notices in storage spaces, or the off-kilter looks traded at the rec center. Be that as it may, for the majority of us, Kegels remain covered in secret - a place that is known for awkward presses and sketchy viability.

Indeed, fellas, I'm here to let you know there's an entire neglected side to Kegels, a side that is not just about essential fixing and holding. Enter the domain of quick Kegels, a unique advantage for anybody looking to open another degree of control and endurance in the room.

Presently, before we plunge into the low down, how about we address the obvious issue at hand: distrust. Trust me, I've been there. My underlying introduction to Kegels felt like a weak effort to press a maverick volleyball that wouldn't move. However at that point, I coincidentally found the idea of quick Kegels, and tried to keep your hat on, it was a disclosure.

Consider a quick Kegel a fast fire constriction of your pelvic floor muscles. It resembles a progression of fast "flicks" down there, zeroing in on speed and accuracy as opposed to a supported hold. It could sound basic, however dominating this procedure can be an excursion of self-revelation and, might I venture to say, a dash of strengthening.

Here's the reason I'm a particularly immense supporter for quick Kegels:

Building Endurance is a Long distance race, Not a Run: We should be genuine, conventional Kegels can get tiring, quick. Holding a withdrawal for broadened periods can leave you feeling exhausted and deterred. Quick Kegels, then again, permit you to fabricate perseverance by consolidating short, fast constrictions into your daily practice. It resembles preparing your pelvic floor muscles for a speedy eruption of movement, which is exactly what you want for maximized execution in the room.

Control Becomes the dominant focal point: Envision yourself exploring a winding mountain street - that is the sort of exact control you can accomplish with quick Kegels. These fast compressions assist you with leveling up your skill to draw in and discharge your pelvic floor muscles rapidly. In the room, this means better command over-excitement and discharge, permitting you to broaden joy for both yourself and your accomplice.

(Monotony wears on the soul Kegel Schedules): Can we just be real, doing likewise Kegel practice all day, every day can get dreary. Quick Kegels add an entirely different layer of energy to your everyday practice. They're a great method for testing yourself and keep things fascinating. Furthermore, consolidating them close by customary Kegels makes a balanced exercise for your pelvic floor, focusing on both strength and perseverance.

Past the Room: The advantages of quick Kegels reach out a long way past those hot room meetings. Fortifying your pelvic floor muscles with this procedure can further develop bladder control, lessening the feared releases that can torment men as we age. It can likewise prompt better center dependability and stance, leaving you feeling more certain and empowered over the course of the day.

In any case, stand by, there's something else! Here are a few functional tips to assist you with excelling at the quick Kegel:

Tracking down Your Stream: Very much like any activity, it's vital to confine the right muscles prior to making a plunge. The work of art "pee stop" method is an incredible beginning stage. Whenever you've recognized those slippery pelvic floor muscles, you can start rehearsing fast withdrawals. Envision pressing a pea, not a grapefruit.

Begin Slow, Go Consistent: Don't be a legend! Start with short arrangements of 5-10 quick Kegels, zeroing in on structure as opposed to speed. As you gain certainty, continuously increment the quantity of redundancies and sets. Keep in mind, consistency is key here. Go for the gold sets over the course of the day, integrated into your current daily practice.

Slow Kegels: Building Strength and Endurance

Can we just be real, folks. We as a whole need that handy solution, that moment satisfaction. It applies to everything, isn't that so? Exercises, feasts, even...well, you understand everything. In any case, with regards to Kegels, in all actuality, without rushing genuinely comes out on top in the race.

I know, I know. You may be envisioning vast arrangements of dreary presses, addressing assuming that anything is in any event, occurring down there. However, trust me, the force of slow Kegels is an unlikely treasure ready to be uncovered. It's an excursion, not a run, and the prizes are certainly worth the venture.

Here is what I've realized: the underlying energy of Kegels can rapidly blur assuming we center exclusively around speed and force. We hold and deliver, expecting to see prompt outcomes, just to be left inclination disappointed and uncertain. Yet, here's the clear-cut advantage - slow Kegels. It could sound unreasonable, however zeroing in on a conscious, controlled constriction opens an unheard of degree of solidarity and perseverance in your pelvic floor.

Think about it like this. Envision attempting to construct a block facade. You could erratically toss blocks together, expecting a speedy construction. In any case, couldn't a painstakingly built wall, every block carefully positioned, be undeniably more steady and enduring? That is the pith of slow Kegels. You're not simply crushing; you're developing an underpinning of fortitude starting from the earliest stage.

This is the way it changed my own Kegel experience:

1. Uncovering the Secret Profundities: Can we just be real for a minute, a large portion of us have an unclear comprehension of our pelvic floor muscles. We could know they're "down there" some place, however genuinely interfacing with them can be a test. Slow Kegels turned into my vital aspect for opening this secret world. By zeroing in on a sluggish, controlled constriction, I could really feel the unobtrusive commitment profound inside. It was a disclosure, a newly discovered consciousness of an essential piece of my body.

2. Developing Fortitude More than ever: Fail to remember the short lived consumption of speedy presses. Slow Kegels resemble a gradual process that develops veritable fortitude. Envision holding a board - it doesn't feel like much from the beginning, yet as you stand firm on the situation, your center begins to shout. That is the sorcery of slow Kegels. By holding the withdrawal for a supported period, you're constraining your pelvic floor muscles to work harder, developing genuine fortitude and perseverance.

3. Endurance You Can Feel: At any point feel like your "battery" runs out excessively rapidly? Definitely, me as well. In any case, slow Kegels have been a unique advantage. By zeroing in on controlled withdrawals, I've seen a critical improvement in my general endurance. It makes an interpretation of the room (wink, wink), yet additionally to all that I do. From longer exercises to just climbing steps without feeling short of breath, the advantages are obvious.

4. Certainty with Each Crush: Perhaps the most unforeseen advantage of slow Kegels has been the certainty help. It could sound weird, however zeroing in on my pelvic floor wellbeing has provided me with a freshly discovered feeling of control and mindfulness. It resembles realizing you've invested the hard effort, constructed a strong groundwork, and are prepared to take on whatever comes your direction. A calm certainty emanates from the back to front.

All in all, how would you really get everything rolling with slow Kegels? Here are a few hints:

- **See as Your Base:** Before you jump into slow Kegels, it's essential to distinguish your pelvic floor muscles. The work of art "stop pee stream" procedure works for some, yet make sure to analyze. Rests, unwind, and attempt to fix the muscles around your private parts and butt. You ought to feel an unpretentious lift.

- **Unwavering mindsets always win in the end:** Whenever you've distinguished your muscles, center around sluggish, controlled compressions. Hold back nothing crush for 5-10 seconds, then deliver it totally. Rehash this for 10-15 redundancies, bit by bit expanding the hold time as you get more grounded.

- **Inhale Simple:** Don't pause your breathing! Legitimate breathing is fundamental for compelling Kegels. Breathe in as you unwind, and breathe out as you contract. This guarantees you're not stressing and considers ideal muscle commitment.

- **Consistency is Vital:** Like any activity, consistency is critical. Hold back nothing a couple of sets of slow Kegels day to day. You can coordinate them into your daily practice - while staring at the television, perusing, or in any event, holding up in line. The magnificence is, they should be possible anyplace.

Leveling Up Your Kegel Game: Advanced Techniques for Experienced Men

---

Weighted Kegel Exercises: Adding Resistance for Increased Challenge

Can we just be real, folks. The universe of Kegel activities can feel a little… tame. We press, we hold, we rehash. Viable, sure, however where's the test? Where's the feeling of achievement that accompanies propelling ourselves past our usual ranges of familiarity? Indeed, my companions, this is where weighted Kegels enter the image, prepared to change your daily practice from "that is old news" to an all out center odyssey.

Presently, before you imagine yourself raising free weights down there (trust me, that is not the picture we're going for), we should unload the universe of weighted Kegel works out. Everything no doubt revolves around adding a hint of protection from your standard Kegel schedule, presenting another degree of challenge that will have your pelvic floor muscles singing (OK, perhaps not singing, yet certainly feeling the consume positively).

Yet, consider this: the choice to integrate weighted Kegels ought not be messed with. It's anything but a one-size-fits-all suggestion. Think about it like adding loads to your bicep twists - you couldn't bounce directly to a 50-pound hand weight, okay? The equivalent goes for Kegels. We really want to construct an establishment, and expert the nuts and bolts, prior to wandering into the universe of weighted obstruction.

Thus, assuming you've been perseveringly doing your standard Kegels for some time and are feeling that tingle to drive yourself further, then, at that point, this section is for you. Think of it as your own personal guide to the universe of weighted Kegels, perfect with a solid portion of support, a sprinkle of wariness, and a ton of "no need to relive that" insight.

Can we just look at things objectively? Standard Kegels can turn into a little... daily schedule. We fall into a mood, a safe place, and keeping in mind that viable, it can come up short in a flash of fervor. Weighted Kegels, my companions, once again introduce that test. They force your pelvic floor muscles to work harder, adjust, and develop further.

Consider it along these lines. Envision yourself going to the rec center interestingly. You can lift those 5-pound loads the entire day, however in the long run, your body changes. To continue to see improvement, you want to build the obstruction. Weighted Kegels work the same way. They push your pelvic floor muscles past their ongoing capacities, prompting expanded strength, perseverance, and at last, an unheard of degree of control.

Be that as it may, the advantages reach out a long way past the physical. Weighted Kegels can likewise be a significant certainty sponsor. Dominating this seriously difficult type of Kegels can unbelievably enable. It's a demonstration of your devotion, your obligation to propelling yourself, and at last, to assuming command over your wellbeing and prosperity.

The Profound Rollercoaster: From Incredulity to Fulfillment

Presently, I'll be quick to concede, I wasn't generally a devotee to weighted Kegels. In the same way as other of you, I began with the essentials, run of the mill press and hold. Also, you will scarcely believe, it requires an investment to get results. There were snapshots of uncertainty, of addressing whether I was in any event, doing them right. However, gradually, consistently, I began to feel a distinction. My control improved, my endurance expanded, and we should simply express, things in the room turned into significantly more… fulfilling (for both me and my accomplice).

Then, at that point, I coincidentally found the idea of weighted Kegels. Fascinated, yet in addition somewhat distrustful, I chose to check them out. The initial not many endeavors… indeed, how about we simply say it wasn't pretty. Tracking down the right weight, and the right inclusion strategy, all took some training. In any case, there was a flash, a feeling of challenge that pushed me along.

And afterward, it clicked. I figured out the perfect balance, that ideal mix of weight and control. The sensation of my pelvic floor muscles staying at work past 40 hours, adjusting to the new interest, it was... stimulating. It was a demonstration of my commitment, a sign that I was driving myself higher than ever (play on words expected). In any case, the genuine award came later, in the room. The expanded control, the elevated endurance - it improved things significantly. How about we simply express, the two of us were left inclination more associated, and more fulfilled than any time in recent memory.

Diving in: A Manual for Exploring Weighted Kegels

Okay, so you're captivated. Taking your Kegel routine to a higher level has provoked your curiosity. Be that as it may, where
Where do you try to start? Listen to this: wandering into the universe of weighted Kegels requires a mindful and estimated approach. It's anything but a rush to the end goal, yet an excursion of investigation and revelation. This are a few critical contemplations to remember:

Ace the Rudiments First: This can't be focused sufficiently on. Before considering weighted Kegels, guarantee you've dominated the standard Kegel procedure. This implies having the option to disconnect and agree with your pelvic floor muscles really. On the off chance that you're uncertain, counsel an actual specialist or medical care proficient for direction.

Begin Light and Slowly Increment: Recollect the similarity of bicep twists? A similar guideline applies here. Try not to get the heaviest-weighted Kegel available at the very first moment. Start with a lightweight, something that gives delicate opposition without stressing your pelvic floor muscles. As your solidarity and control improve, you can build your weight bit by bit.

Pay attention to Your Body: This is vital. Weighted Kegels ought to never cause agony or uneasiness. On the off chance that you experience any aggravation, stop right away and counsel a medical care proficient. Focus on your body's signs, and change the weight or strategy likewise.

View as the Right Fit: Weighted Kegels come in different structures, from weighted cones to silicone balls. Investigation and find what feels generally great for you. There's no "one size fits all" arrangement - focus on solace and convenience.

Consistency is Critical: Very much like with standard Kegels, consistency is pivotal for progress. Hold back nothing sets of weighted Kegel practices each day, regardless of whether it's only for a couple of moments. Keep in mind, it's about better standards without ever compromising. Center around appropriate structure and controlled withdrawals.

Embrace the Excursion: Weighted Kegels are an excursion, not an objective. There will be snapshots of dissatisfaction, of scrutinizing your advancement. In any case, don't surrender! Center around the little triumphs, the steady upgrades in strength and control. Commend your commitment, and the outcomes will ultimately follow.

The Rewards Await: Beyond the Physical Benefits
Let's talk about the payoff. Weighted Kegels aren't just about building more grounded pelvic floor muscles (albeit that is a really wonderful advantage in itself). They can prompt a fountain of beneficial outcomes, both genuinely and inwardly.

Upgraded Sexual Execution: More grounded, more controlled pelvic floor muscles can altogether work on sexual execution for the two men and their accomplices. Expanded endurance, better control, and elevated awareness - these are expected advantages of integrating weighted Kegels into your daily schedule.

Further developed Bladder Control: Feeble pelvic floor muscles can add to urinary incontinence. Fortifying these muscles with weighted Kegels can prompt better bladder control, decreasing the gamble of humiliating breaks.

Certainty Lift: Dominating a difficult activity like weighted Kegels can staggeringly enable. It's a demonstration of your devotion, your obligation to personal development, and at last, your capacity to assume responsibility for your wellbeing and prosperity.

<u>A Last Note: You Got This!</u>

See, I get it. Weighted Kegels could appear to be threatening from the start. However, trust me, they're an unimaginable instrument for taking your Kegel routine to a higher level. With devotion, tolerance, and a sound portion of self-revelation, you can open a universe of advantages, both physical and profound. Anyway, would you say you are prepared to go all in? Keep in mind, you have this! Embrace the test, praise the excursion, and experience the fulfillment that accompanies stretching your boundaries. Your body, and your accomplice, will thank you for it.

Biofeedback Training: Receiving Real-Time Feedback on Your Technique

Can we just be real for a moment, folks. Kegels can be a confounding excursion. We press, we hold, we trust we're getting things done as needs be. Be that as it may, a pestering uncertainty frequently waits: would we say we are really focusing on the right muscles? Is it true or not that we are investing the energy, however coming up short completely? This, my companions, is where biofeedback preparing steps in, prepared to focus a light on the secret universe of your pelvic floor.

Envision having a fitness coach, not so much for your biceps or abs, but rather for the most critical (and frequently ignored) muscle bunch in your center - your pelvic floor. Biofeedback preparing offers precisely that. A progressive methodology gives constant input on your Kegel strategy, changing the demonstration of getting into an interesting excursion of self-revelation.

Presently, before you imagine some cutting edge contraption joined to… indeed, how about we simply say delicate regions… unwind. Biofeedback preparing comes in different structures, some more careful than others. In any case, the fundamental guideline continues as before: to give objective information on your pelvic floor muscle movement, enabling you to refine your strategy and open the genuine capability of your center.

<u>The Suspicious Me: From Uncertainty to Interest</u>

I admit I wasn't generally a biofeedback advocate. For quite a long time, I depended on standard Kegel crush, staying cautiously optimistic. However, can we just be real for a minute, the outcomes were… dubious. There was consistently that annoying uncertainty, whether or not I was genuinely captivating the right muscles.

Then, I coincidentally found biofeedback preparing. Captivated, yet additionally somewhat wary, I chose to check it out. The main meeting was… educational, most definitely. The biofeedback specialist made sense of how a little sensor would be set either remotely (on the perineum) or inside (through the butt or vagina) contingent upon the sort of biofeedback utilized. This sensor would then communicate signs to a screen, showing my pelvic floor muscle action progressively.

<u>Lights, Camera, Kegels! : The Biofeedback Experience</u>

Okay, the genuine biofeedback experience wasn't so sensational as a Hollywood film debut. However, it was absolutely entrancing. As I performed Kegels, the screen showed lines and charts, a visual portrayal of my muscle action. Interestingly, I could see the distinction among stressing and genuine pelvic floor muscle commitment.

The advisor directed me through different activities, assisting me with understanding the subtleties of various Kegel procedures - slow presses, quick heartbeats, and in the middle between. They gave continuous input, empowering me to change my stance, my breathing, and in particular, my Kegel procedure.

Past the Signal: Profound Leap forwards

In any case, the advantages of biofeedback preparation stretched out a long ways past the blares and lines on the screen. It was a close to home excursion too. Interestingly, I felt a feeling of command over my pelvic floor. The dissatisfaction of vulnerability, of not knowing whether I was getting everything done well, started to blur. Biofeedback engaged me to assume responsibility, to turn into a functioning member in my own prosperity.

It wasn't just about fortifying my pelvic floor, albeit that was surely a reward. It was about self-disclosure, about acquiring a more profound comprehension of my body and its capacities. This freshly discovered mindfulness converted into a newly discovered certainty, both in the exercise center and then some.

<u>A Universe of Potential outcomes: The Advantages of Biofeedback Preparing</u>

Biofeedback preparation offers a huge number of advantages that reach out a long way past the underlying "goodness" factor. Here are only a couple of justifications for why you should seriously mull over checking it out:

Further developed Kegel Procedure: Biofeedback gives constant criticism, guaranteeing you're focusing on the right muscles with the right power. No seriously speculating, simply unadulterated, pure viability.

Quicker Results: Seeing your muscle movement on a screen can essentially speed up your advancement. Biofeedback assists you with refining your procedure rapidly, prompting quicker and more observable outcomes.

Upgraded Inspiration: Can we just be real, staying with Kegels can be intense. Biofeedback preparing infuses a portion of fervor into everyday practice. Seeing your improvement on the screen can be unimaginably rousing, filling your obligation to long haul results.

Tending to Explicit Circumstances: Biofeedback preparing can be an important device in overseeing different circumstances, including urinary incontinence, erectile brokenness, and pelvic agony. With the assistance of a prepared specialist, you can foster a designated program to address your particular necessities.

Is Biofeedback Ideal for You? Going with an Educated Choice

Biofeedback preparation isn't a great fit for everybody. It probably won't be promptly accessible in all areas, and protection inclusion can shift.

Chapter 7: Kegel Exercises and Erectile Dysfunction: A Potential Ally

Understanding Erectile Dysfunction and Its Causes

We should discuss something men seldom discuss - erectile brokenness (ED). An expression can strike dread into the core of even the most certain person. I know in light of the fact that, for some time there, ED was my unwanted friend. It was anything but a consistent presence, however those periodic snapshots of... disappointment... left me feeling like an emptied swell, the demeanor of certainty whooshing out of me quicker than I could say "closeness."

Perhaps you're gesturing your head at the present time, a quiet affirmation of a battle you assumed you were separated from everyone else in. Trust me, you're not. ED is surprisingly normal, influencing a great many men around the world. However, that doesn't make it any simpler to manage.

Listen to this: dealing with ED directly can be terrifying. There's the underlying shock, the scrutinizing, the apprehension that your sexual coexistence - and perhaps your manliness - is finished. In any case, before you surrender to an existence of darkened lights and off-kilter quiets, we should dive into the universe of ED, figure out its causes, and in particular, investigate the way back to recovering your certainty.

The Close to home Rollercoaster: From Frustration to Assurance

Whenever it first worked out, I was walloped. There was the underlying disarray, the mishandling endeavor to rescue what is happening, and afterward the devastating influx of disillusionment. It wasn't just about the actual angle - it was the catastrophe for my self image, the insecurity that came crashing down on me. Is it true or not that I was broken? Is it true or not that I was as of now not a man?

Those underlying inquiries were dim, and loaded up with self-question. Be that as it may, gradually, an alternate inclination arose - assurance. I wouldn't allowED to characterize myself, to take my certainty, or to direct my sexual coexistence. In this way, I began digging, exploring all that I could about the condition. Also, learn to expect the unexpected. There was a good reason to have hope.

Figuring out the Adversary: Demystifying the Reasons for ED

ED isn't a sickness, yet a side effect of a basic issue. It's a warning, a sign that something's not exactly right. The causes can be physical, mental, or a blend of both. Here are a portion of the primary guilty parties:

Actual Causes: These can go from vascular issues (diminished blood stream to the penis) to hormonal irregular characteristics (low testosterone levels) to nerve harm (from diabetes or medical procedure). Certain prescriptions can likewise add to ED.

Mental Causes: Stress, tension, execution pressure, sorrow - this multitude of close to home variables can assume a critical part in erectile brokenness. At times, a terrible involvement with the room can prompt a pattern of uneasiness, making future experiences considerably more troublesome.

Ending the Quietness: Conversing with Your Primary care physician (and Perhaps Your Accomplice)

This is where things can get precarious. Men, can we just be real, we're not precisely known for discussing our sexual battles. Be that as it may, stop and think for a minute: ED is an ailment, and very much like some other clinical issue, it should be tended to. Conversing with your PCP could feel humiliating at first, yet trust me, they've heard everything previously. They have the information and skill to assist you with getting to the underlying driver of your ED and foster a treatment plan.

Also, here's another significant discussion - the one with your accomplice. Open correspondence is vital in any relationship, particularly with regards to closeness. Conversing with your accomplice about your ED can be terrifying, but on the other hand it's a potential chance to interface, share your weaknesses, and track down help. Keep in mind, they're probably similarly as confused and stressed as you seem to be.

The Way to Recuperation: Treatment Choices and the Force of Inspiration

1. **The uplifting news?** ED is treatable. There's an entire weapons store of choices accessible, contingent upon the hidden reason. Here are a few likely methodologies:
2. **Way of life Changes:** Exercise, solid eating routine, stress the board - these way of life changes can fundamentally affect your general wellbeing, including your sexual wellbeing.

3. **Prescriptions:** There are different drugs accessible that can assist with further developing bloodstream to the penis or address hormonal awkward nature.
4. **Treatment:** Assuming mental variables are at play, treatment can be extraordinarily useful in overseeing pressure, uneasiness, or execution pressure.
5. **Vacuum Siphons and Embeds:** These are further developed treatment choices for men who haven't answered well to different methodologies.

It's a Long distance race, Not a Run: Keeping up with Progress and Embracing Closeness

The way to overseeing ED is a drawn out obligation to your wellbeing and prosperity. Try not to anticipate an enchanted pill or a handy solution. Treating ED takes time, persistence, and a readiness to examine and find what turns out best for you. Be that as it may, here's what is significant: you don't need to go through this by itself. There are assets accessible, support bunches you can associate with, and medical care experts who are there to direct you constantly.

Something other than Sex: Recovering Closeness and Rediscovering Certainty

Can we just look at things objectively for a moment, ED can create a shaded area over your whole relationship.

The feeling of dread toward disappointment, and the pressure of execution - these variables can negatively affect closeness. However, recollecting closeness is about far beyond sex. It's about association, about profound closeness, about feeling cherished and wanted. Center around those parts of your relationship - the snuggles, the common chuckling, the profound discussions. Closeness doesn't need to be exclusively characterized by infiltration. Investigate alternate ways of associating with your accomplice, to feel wanted, and to rediscover the delight of actual touch.

The Reason to have some hope: A More promising time to come Is standing by

Confronting ED can be a pivotal occasion. It tends to be an impetus for assuming responsibility for your wellbeing, for focusing on your prosperity, and for cultivating open correspondence inside your relationship. The excursion may not be simple, however the prizes are huge. By grasping the reasons for ED, looking for proficient assistance, and focusing on a drawn out approach, you can recover your certainty, rediscover closeness, and at last, compose another part in your sexual wellbeing story.

A Last Note: You Are In good company

Keep in mind, a large number of men overall experience ED. It's a typical condition, yet it doesn't need to characterize you. There's trust, there's help, and there's a way back to a satisfying sexual coexistence. In this way, take a full breath, accumulate your boldness, and venture out toward recovering your certainty. You have this!

The Potential Role of Kegel Exercises in Erectile Dysfunction Management

---

We should discuss something men seldom utter resoundingly - erectile brokenness (ED). An expression can leave you feeling like a flattened inflatable, the demeanor of certainty whooshing out quicker than you can say "closeness." I know. For some time there, ED was a shadow prowling at the edges of my relationship, projecting a long and unwanted uncertainty over my manliness.

The underlying shock is ruthless - the mistake, oneself doubting, the trepidation that your sexual coexistence is finished. Yet, before you surrender to an existence of diminished lights and abnormal quiet, we should investigate a likely way to recover control: Kegel works out.

Past the Dissatisfaction: A Flash of Trust and a Doubtful Psyche

OK, when I originally caught wind of Kegels as a likely weapon against ED, I'll just let it out - I had misgivings. Gripping a few secretive muscles down there didn't precisely seem like a fight plan for room predominance. Yet, listen to this: I was frantic. Ready to take a stab at anything to recover that flash, that trust in the room. In this way, I dove recklessly into the universe of Kegels, a combination of trust and wariness whirling in my stomach.

Disclosing the Force to be reckoned with Underneath Figuring out Your Pelvic Floor

Before we dive into the universe of Kegel works out, we should discuss the secret force to be reckoned with underneath everything - your pelvic floor muscles. Consider them a lounger, supporting your bladder, rectum, and - you got it - your erection. Solid pelvic floor muscles add to bladder control as well as assume an essential part in accomplishing and keeping an erection.

The Science Behind the Crush: How Kegels Could Assist with ED

Here's where things get fascinating. Erection is about blood stream. When excited, blood races to the penis, filling elastic chambers and making it solidify. Powerless pelvic floor muscles can obstruct this blood stream, blocking your capacity to accomplish or keep an erection. This is where Kegel practices come in. By reinforcing these muscles, you might possibly:

- **Further develop Blood Stream:** More grounded muscles mean better blood stream all through the pelvic area, possibly expanding bloodstream to the penis during excitement.
- **Upgraded Control:** Kegels can work on your command over the muscles engaged with erection, permitting you to keep a firmer erection for longer.
- **Elevated Sensation:** Standard Kegel practice can increment responsiveness in the penis, prompting a seriously satisfying sexual experience.

<u>The Doubter's Excursion: My Involvement in Kegels</u>

Presently, we should get genuine. Kegels are certainly not an enchanted pill. They require devotion, consistency, and a sound portion of persistence. The initial not many weeks were... uninteresting. Is it true or not that I was treating them terribly? Was each of the monster self-influenced consequences? However at that point, gradually, I began to feel a distinction. My erections felt firmer, more maintained. There was a newly discovered control, a feeling of responsibility over my body that had been absent for some time.

It's Not Just About You: The Profound Effect on Connections

We should not fail to remember the profound part of ED. It's not just about the actual demonstration of sex - it's about closeness, association, and feeling wanted by your accomplice. At the point when ED strikes, it can make a wedge in your relationship, pushing you and your accomplice separated. In any case, consider this: when you begin to see improvement with Kegels, in addition to your erections improve - it's your certainty. You stroll into the room with your head held high, prepared to interface with your accomplice on a more profound level. What's more, that, old buddy, can significantly affect your relationship.

A Delicate Update: Kegels Aren't an Independent Arrangement

While Kegels can be an integral asset in overseeing ED, it's memorable and vital they probably won't be the main arrangement required.

Here's the reason:

- **Figuring out the Reason:** ED has different causes, from actual issues like diabetes or low testosterone to mental elements like pressure and nervousness. Tending to the underlying driver is urgent for long haul achievement.

- **Counsel a Medical care Proficient:** Don't hesitate for even a moment to converse with your PCP. They can analyze the reason for your ED and suggest a customized treatment plan that could incorporate way of life changes, medicine, or even treatment.
- **A Multi-Pronged Methodology:** Join Kegel practices with other solid propensities like activity, a reasonable eating regimen, and stress the executives for a comprehensive way to deal with overseeing ED.

Past the Room: The Startling Advantages of Kegel Power

Can we just look at things objectively for a minute, more grounded erections are a really convincing motivation to embrace Kegel works out. However, the advantages stretch out a long way past the room. Here are a few surprising ways Kegel power can improve your general prosperity:

Further developed Bladder Control: Powerless pelvic floor muscles can add to urinary incontinence, those humiliating releases that can disturb your regular routine. More grounded pelvic floor muscles, on account of normal Kegel practice, can altogether further develop bladder control.

Upgraded Sexual Endurance: Kegels don't simply help erections - they can likewise work on sexual endurance. More grounded pelvic floor muscles permit you to keep up with control during intercourse for longer, prompting a seriously satisfying encounter for both you and your accomplice.

A Certainty Lift: Dominating Kegel works out, an apparently straightforward yet testing task, can staggeringly enable. It's a demonstration of your devotion, your obligation to assume responsibility for your wellbeing, and at last, your capacity to recover command over your body.

Keep in mind, You're In good company: A Last Note of Consolation

ED is a typical issue, influencing a great many men around the world. It may very well be a baffling and segregating experience, yet you don't need to go through this by itself. There are assets accessible, medical services experts who can help, and a local area of men who figure out your battle. Furthermore, in particular, there's trust. Kegel activities may be a piece of the riddle, a device in your stockpile for recapturing control. In this way, embrace the excursion, praise the little triumphs, and recollect, a more grounded pelvic floor prompts a more sure, satisfying you, both all through the room.

Strengthening Pelvic Floor Muscles for Improved Blood Flow

We should discuss a piece of your body that frequently gets eclipsed - the pelvic floor. Not precisely a point rules supper discussions, but rather trust me, this secret stalwart assumes an essential part in your general wellbeing and prosperity. For my purposes, it was an excursion of disclosure, a disclosure that went a long way past the room and into the domain of feeling areas of strength for those really in charge.

Perhaps you've heard murmurs regarding pelvic floor works out (Kegels, anybody?) and their alleged advantages. Or on the other hand perhaps you're encountering a few pestering issues - urinary spillage, a debilitated center, or even erectile brokenness (ED). Whatever your justification behind wandering into this region, welcome on board. We should dive into the universe of reinforcing your pelvic floor muscles, and open a universe of advantages that stretch out a long way past what you could at first envision.

<u>From Dissatisfaction to Interest: A Reminder and a Journey for Replies</u>

For a really long time, I overlooked the unobtrusive clues my body was sending. A periodic post-exercise "release," the sensation of a center that wasn't exactly basically areas of strength for as it used to be - I dismissed them as minor disturbances. However at that point, things went ahead. An apparently innocuous sniffle transformed into a public humiliation, and the dissatisfaction rose over. Something needed to change.

That is the point at which I coincidentally found the idea of the pelvic floor. This organization of muscles supports your bladder, rectum, and contraceptive organs, going about as a crucial emotionally supportive network for your whole center. Also, prepare to be blown away. Feeble pelvic floor muscles could be the offender behind my hardships. Out of nowhere, those murmurs regarding Kegels didn't appear to be so senseless any longer.

The Force of Blood Stream: Energizing Your Body for Ideal Execution

Here is the entrancing association between your pelvic floor and your general wellbeing - blood stream. More grounded pelvic floor muscles further develop blood courses all through the pelvic district. Consider it an organization of thruways. Solid "muscles" going about as smooth street surfaces permit blood to stream unreservedly, supporting your organs and tissues. On the other hand, frail pelvic floor muscles resemble stopped up thruways, obstructing blood stream and possibly prompting a fountain of issues.

Past the Releases: The Startling Advantages of Further developed Blood Stream

The advantages of further developed blood stream, because of a more grounded pelvic floor, reach out a long way past forestalling humiliating breaks. Here is a brief look at what you could insight:

Upgraded Center Strength: A solid pelvic floor goes about as an establishment for your center. Further developed blood stream sustains your center muscles, prompting better solidness, stance, and generally speaking strength. Express farewell to that pain-filled back following a difficult day, and hi to a more certain, strong you.

A Supported Sexual coexistence: Blood stream is urgent for a sound sexual coexistence. For men, more grounded pelvic floor muscles can prompt better erections. For ladies, an expanded blood stream can uplift responsiveness and lead to a seriously satisfying sexual experience. It's a mutual benefit for the two accomplices!

Further developed Bladder Control: Spilling isn't simply humiliating, it tends to be a significant burden.

Reinforcing your pelvic floor muscles can essentially further develop bladder control, permitting you to partake in exercises without stress. Envision running, hopping, or snickering without the feeling of dread toward spills - that is the freeing force of areas of strength for a story.

By and large Prosperity: Further developed blood stream can meaningfully affect your whole body. It can feed your organs, help your resistant framework, and even improve your energy levels. Fortifying your pelvic floor muscles isn't just about fixing a particular issue - it's tied in with putting resources into your general prosperity.

The Excursion Starts: Activities, Methods, and a Delicate Update

Presently, we should get down to the bare essential - how would you fortify your pelvic floor muscles? Here are a few vital activities to kick you off:

Kegel Activities: The exemplary on purpose! Contract and loosen up your pelvic floor muscles as though you're attempting to prevent yourself from peeing halfway. Hold for a couple of moments, then discharge. Rehash this a few times each day.

Span Activities: Lie on your back with knees twisted and feet level on the floor. Lift your hips off the ground, connecting with your center and pelvic floor muscles. Hold for a couple of moments, then lower down.

Squats: This full-body practice likewise connects with your pelvic floor muscles. Stand with your feet shoulder-width separated and crouch as though you will sit in a seat. Make sure you keep your back straight and center locked in. Propel yourself back up to the starting position.

Keep in mind: Consistency is Vital

Very much like structure of any muscle, reinforcing your pelvic floor takes time and commitment. Try not to get deterred on the off chance that you don't get results for the time being. Go for the gold arrangements of pelvic floor practices each day, regardless of whether it's only for a couple of moments. Consistency is critical to accomplishing long haul results.

Pay attention to Your Body

While practice is significant, it's essential to pay attention to your body. On the off chance that you experience any aggravation or uneasiness during your activities, stop right away and counsel a medical services proficient. Legitimate method is fundamental to stay away from injury.

Look for Proficient Direction (if necessary)

There's no disgrace in looking for help from a medical care proficient or pelvic floor actual specialist. They can survey your singular necessities, suggest explicit activities, and guarantee you're performing them accurately. This can be particularly useful assuming that you're managing explicit issues like urinary incontinence or post pregnancy recuperation.

An Excursion, Not an Objective

Reinforcing your pelvic floor muscles is an excursion, not an objective. Embrace the cycle, celebrate little triumphs, and partake in the freshly discovered strength and prosperity that accompanies areas of strength for a story. Keep in mind, it's not just about forestalling spills or further developing your sexual coexistence - it's tied in with assuming responsibility for your wellbeing and feeling really enabled from the back to front.

The Focus point: A More grounded You Is standing by

The pelvic floor, frequently neglected and underrated, assumes a crucial part in our general wellbeing. By reinforcing these muscles, you can open a universe of advantages, from further developed blood stream to a more grounded center, and eventually, a more joyful, better you. Thus, take a full breath, press those pelvic floor muscles (only a tad!), and leave on this excursion of self-revelation. Your whole body will appreciate you for it, trust me.

Enhancing Sexual Stamina and Performance

Can we just be real for a moment, folks. Sex is something beyond the firecrackers finale. It's the common closeness, the profound association, and the gradual process that prompts a fantastic peak for the two accomplices. In any case, consider this: when endurance winds down, that gradual process can flame out excessively rapidly, leaving both of you feeling disheartened and disappointed. Trust me, I've been there. Those snapshots of blurring perseverance can leave you feeling deficient, scrutinizing your manliness, and longing for a method for recapturing control.

However, dread not, individual voyagers on the way to closeness! Improving sexual endurance and execution isn't tied in with pursuing some legendary ideal of "enduring everlastingly." It's tied in with making a seriously satisfying encounter for you as well as your accomplice, broadening that flavorful expectation and shared joy. Furthermore, the uplifting news? There are an entire host of approaches you can investigate, from way of life changes to room procedures, to changing yourself into a sexual endurance machine (indeed, perhaps not a machine, but rather you understand).

From Disillusionment to Assurance: A Flash Lights the Excursion

Whenever it first worked out, I was surprised. The underlying fervor, the structure expectation - and afterward, a disappointingly quick end. It wasn't just about the actual angle - it was the personal effect. The sensation of letting my accomplice down, of neglecting to satisfy some implicit assumption, weighed vigorously on me. However, rather than capitulating to demoralization, a flash of assurance lighted inside. I would not allow this to characterize me, to create a shaded area over my sexual coexistence. Thus, I began digging, exploring all that I could about upgrading sexual endurance. Also, prepare to be blown away. There was a mother lode of data simply ready to be found.

Figuring out the Adversary: The Variables that Impact Endurance

Sexual endurance isn't just about actual ability. It's a complicated transaction of physical, profound, and mental variables. Here are a portion of the central participants:

Actual Wellness: Normal activity further develops blood stream all through the body, including the privates. A solid cardiovascular framework means better perseverance, in the exercise center, yet additionally in the room.

Solid Eating routine: Sustaining your body with entire food varieties gives it the energy and endurance it requires to ideally work. Ditch the handled garbage and embrace an eating regimen wealthy in organic products, vegetables, and lean protein.

Stress The board: Persistent pressure can unleash devastation on your charisma and endurance. Tracking down solid ways of overseeing pressure, whether it's contemplation, exercise, or investing energy in nature, can improve things significantly.

Lack of sleep: Being restless destroys your actual energy as well as dulls your psychological concentration and profound association. Focus on quality rest for ideal sexual execution.

Execution Tension: The strain to perform can be a significant mood killer and an endurance executioner. Center around partaking in the occasion, associating with your accomplice, and relinquishing assumptions.

Past the Rudiments: Room Strategies for Upgraded Pleasure

Now that we've handled the primary components, we should dig into some room strategies that can assist you with broadening the delight and amplify your endurance:

The Specialty of Foreplay: Foreplay isn't just about actual excitement. It's tied in with building expectation, and close to home association, and permitting your body to steadily become stirred. Dial back, investigate each other's bodies, and relish the excursion.

Openness is Absolutely vital: Converse with your accomplice! Open correspondence about your requirements and wants can assist you with fitting your methodology and make a seriously satisfying encounter for both of you.

Center around Strategy: Investigate various positions and procedures that can assist you with keeping an erection and draw out the joy. There's no one size-fits-all methodology - trial and find what turns out best for yourself as well as your accomplice.

Begin Stop Strategy: This is an incredible method for building excitement and control. Animate each other to the place of close to peak, then interruption and spotlight on different types of touch. Rehash this interaction, permitting your excitement to fabricate bit by bit and postpone climax.

Keep in mind, It's an Excursion, Not an Objective

Here is the key important point: upgrading sexual endurance is an excursion, not an objective. It's tied in with embracing sound propensities, cultivating open correspondence with your accomplice, and moving toward sex with a feeling of investigation and happiness. There will be knocks along the street, snapshots of disappointment and self-question. Yet, by zeroing in on the excursion, on making a seriously satisfying encounter for both of you, you'll find a universe of joy and association that goes a long way past, essentially enduring longer. Thus, take a full breath, let go of assumptions, and leave on this thrilling excursion with your accomplice. You may be amazed at the inconceivable encounters ready to be found.

A Last Note: When to Look for Proficient Assistance

While there are numerous things you can do all alone to improve sexual endurance, there are times when expert assistance may be fundamental. In the event that you're encountering constant weariness, erectile brokenness, or determined execution nervousness, think about conversing with a specialist or advisor. They can assist you with recognizing any basic ailments and foster a customized plan to address your interests.

Keep in mind, a sound sexual coexistence is a significant piece of a satisfying relationship. By assuming responsibility for your physical and mental prosperity, and by transparently speaking with your accomplice, you can make a universe of closeness and shared delight that goes a long way past endurance. Presently go forward, investigate, and partake in the excursion!

Important Considerations: When to Consult a Doctor Regarding Erectile Dysfunction

---

We should discuss something men seldom utter so anyone might hear - erectile brokenness (ED). An expression can leave you feeling like an emptied expand, the demeanor of certainty whooshing out quicker than you can say "closeness." I know the inclination. For some time there, ED was a shadow prowling at the edges of my relationship, projecting a long and unwanted uncertainty over my manliness.

The underlying shock is fierce - the failure, oneself doubting, the apprehension that your sexual coexistence is finished. Be that as it may, before you surrender to an existence of darkened lights and off-kilter hushes, there's an essential choice to be made: when to counsel a specialist.

The Battle Among Disgrace and Looking for Help: A Man's Interior Fight

Can we just be real, men aren't precisely known for exposing their profound spirits, particularly with regards to something as private as ED. There's a feeling of dread toward judgment, a lost feeling of disgrace, a voice inside that tells you to "intense it out," to imagine all is well. I fought with that voice for some time. The prospect of conversing with a specialist about my failure to perform was embarrassing. However, stop and think for a minute: disregarding the issue won't make it vanish. As a matter of fact, it can have an expanding influence, influencing your relationship, your confidence, and, surprisingly, your general wellbeing.

Past the Physical: The Close to home Cost of ED

ED isn't just about the actual demonstration of sex. It's about closeness, association, and feeling wanted by your accomplice. At the point when ED strikes, it can make a wedge in your relationship, pushing you and your accomplice separated. You could pull out inwardly, dreading closeness will prompt another mistake. Your accomplice could feel befuddled, dismissed, or even inquiry your fascination with them. The close to home cost can be huge, letting you feel confined and be.

Exposing the Foe: Perceiving Signs You Shouldn't Overlook

While a periodic "off night" is totally ordinary, there are a few indications of ED that warrant a specialist's visit. These are a few warnings to watch out for:

Persevering Trouble Getting or Keeping an Erection: This is the clearest side effect, yet it's critical to take note of that intermittent events don't be guaranteed to require clinical consideration. In any case, in the event that it's occurring oftentimes, now is the ideal time to look for proficient assistance.

Diminished Sexual Longing: An unexpected lessening in your drive could be an indication of a basic ailment, for example, low testosterone levels or gloom.

Inconvenience Arriving at Climax: While ED principally connects with erection issues, trouble arriving at climax can likewise be a side effect.

Difficult Erections: On the off chance that your erections are joined by agony or distress, it's essential to counsel a specialist to preclude any fundamental actual issues.

It's Not Just About You: The Effect on Your Accomplice

Keep in mind, ED isn't simply your battle - it influences your accomplice too. They could feel befuddled, disappointed, or even dismissed. Conversing with them straightforwardly and truly about your ED is vital. Tell them you're in good company, that you're looking for help, and that you esteem your relationship.

Venturing out: What's in store from Your Primary care physician

The specialist's office could appear to be an overwhelming possibility, however stop and think for a minute: specialists see this constantly. ED is a typical condition, and they're there to help. This is what's in store:

Open Correspondence: tell the truth and forthright about your side effects. The more data you give, the better your PCP can analyze the reason for your ED.

Actual Assessment: An actual test can assist with distinguishing any fundamental states of being that may be adding to your ED.

Blood Tests: Blood tests can check for hormonal uneven characters, for example, low testosterone, which can add to ED.

Past the Discussion: Treatment Choices and a More promising time to come

The uplifting news? ED is treatable. There's an entire weapons store of choices accessible, contingent upon the fundamental reason. Here are a few possible methodologies:

Way of life Changes: Exercise, solid eating regimen, and stress the board can all decidedly affect your general wellbeing and sexual capability.

Meds: There are different drugs accessible that can assist with further developing bloodstream to the penis or address hormonal awkward nature.

Treatment: On the off chance that mental variables are affecting everything, treatment can be unbelievably useful in overseeing pressure, nervousness, or execution pressure.

Vacuum Siphons and Embeds: These are further developed treatment choices for men who haven't answered well

Recapturing Control, Recovering Closeness: The Excursion to a Satisfying Sexual coexistence

Conversing with a specialist about ED could appear to be an obstacle, however it's the most vital move towards recovering control of your sexual wellbeing and your relationship. Just have this in mind, you're in good company in this. ED is a typical condition, and there's help accessible. With open correspondence with your PCP and accomplice, and an eagerness to investigate treatment choices, you can conquer ED and rediscover the delight of closeness. The street ahead probably won't be simple, however the objective - a satisfying sexual coexistence and a more grounded relationship - is totally worth the excursion.

Chapter 8: Building a Stronger You: Exercises to Complement Your Kegel Routine

Leg Lunges: Engaging Multiple Muscle Groups

We should discuss serious areas of strength for getting. "Great search in a bathing" areas of strength for suit, strong, fit, "overcome any" areas of strength for challenge. Furthermore, the uplifting news is, you needn't bother with an extravagant exercise center participation or a room loaded with costly hardware to accomplish that sort of solidarity. One straightforward yet unquestionably successful activity can change your lower body - the leg rush.

Perhaps you're a novice, feeling a little scared by the weight rack. Or on the other hand maybe you're a carefully prepared rec center participant hoping to change up your daily practice. The leg jump greets you wholeheartedly (or, indeed, solid legs). It's an activity that anybody, paying little heed to wellness level, can integrate into their exercise plan. Also, trust me, the proof is in the pudding.

From Cynic to Devotee: My Excursion with Leg Thrusts

I wasn't generally a thrust lover. As a matter of fact, for quite a while, I saw them as a discipline workout - something coaches held for the people who really considered skipping leg day. However at that point, a savvy companion (and can we just look at things objectively for a minute, a little self-reflection about my dismissed lower body) persuaded me to check them out. Furthermore, try to keep your hat on, it was a disclosure. Lurches weren't just about consuming quads - they were a door to a more grounded center, better equilibrium, and a newly discovered appreciation for the sheer force of my legs.

The Orchestra of Solidarity: The Muscles Took part in a Leg Rush

The excellence of the leg lurch lies in its capacity to draw in numerous muscle bunches at the same time. Here is the symphony playing in your body during an ideal lurch:

Quadriceps (Quads): These are the stalwart muscles on the facade of your thighs. Thrusts work them hard, chiseling and reinforcing them for that conditioned leg look.

Hamstrings: The frequently disregarded muscles on the rear of your thighs get a serious exercise with rushes, further developing adaptability and adding capacity to your developments.

Glutes: Lurches are a glute-building machine! These muscles add to a chiseled rear as well as assume a significant part in soundness and center strength.

Center: Keeping up with legitimate structure during a thrust requires center commitment, reinforcing your center, and working on by and large equilibrium.

Building Your Establishment: A Bit by bit Manual for Dominating the Leg Jump

Now that you're siphoned (quip expected) about the advantages of leg thrusts, we should separate the appropriate structure so you can receive the full benefits. Keep in mind, structure is vital to staying away from injury and expanding viability. This is a bit by bit guide for fledglings:

Stand tall: Begin with your feet hip-width separated and your center locked in. Envision pulling your gut button towards your spine for that additional piece of center security.

Move Forward: Step in the right direction with one leg, arriving with your heel first. An incredible guideline is to make a major stride - generally the distance of a lung assault (albeit ideally, you will not be rushing at anybody!).

Lower Yourself: As you step forward, twist the two knees. Mean to bring down your back knee towards the ground, however don't allow it to contact. Consider keeping your front knee stacked straight over your lower leg for appropriate arrangement.

Propel Yourself Back Up: Connect with your glutes and quads to propel yourself back up to the beginning position. Center around pushing through your front heel for a strong lift.

Rehash and Switch Legs: Whenever you've finished one jump on one leg, rehash the whole movement with the other leg. Hold back the number of redundancies on every leg, bit by bit expanding the number as you get more grounded.

<u>**Favorable to Tips for Novices: Becoming the best at the Rush**</u>

Here are a few extra tips to assist you with idealizing your leg jump procedure:

1. **Keep your Back Straight:** Abstain from slouching your back during the lurch. Keep a tall stance with your center locked in.
2. **Look Forward:** Don't peer down at your feet! Keep your head in accordance with your spine and your look engaged forward.
3. **Inhale Simple:** Make sure to inhale all through the activity. Breathe in as you lower yourself down, and breathe out as you propel yourself back up.
4. **Begin Bodyweight As it were:** As a novice, center around consummating your structure with bodyweight rushes prior to adding loads.
5. **Pay attention to Your Body:** Don't propel yourself excessively hard. In the event that you feel any aggravation, stop the activity and counsel a specialist.
6. **Minor departure from the Exemplary Rush:** Whenever you've dominated the essential lurch, there are numerous varieties you can investigate to target different muscle gatherings or add an additional test. Models incorporate strolling

rushes, invert lurches, side jumps, and Bulgarian split squats.

7. **Adding Weight for Expanded Power:** As you get more grounded, you can steadily build the trouble of your jumps by adding weight. Hand weights, iron weights, or even a weighted vest can be generally consolidated to additional test your muscles.

8. **The Significance of Rest and Recuperation:** Remember the significance of rest and recuperation after an exercise. Give your muscles time to fix and reconstruct, permitting them to develop further for your next thrust meeting.

Plank Variations: Building Core Strength and Stability

We should discuss the center, people. Not the close to home center, albeit that is significant as well, yet the actual center - the stalwart that sits at the focal point of your body. A solid center isn't just about washboard abs (albeit those are a pleasant advantage!). It's about solidness, strength, and the establishment for a sound, torment free life. In any case, can we just be real, customary crunches can get somewhat... all things considered, exhausting. What's more, here and there, you simply need a test, something to drive you further.

That is where board varieties come in. They're like the superheroes of center activities, offering an assorted scope of choices to target various muscles, keep things intriguing, and leave you feeling like you've really vanquished your exercise. Furthermore, trust me, the sensation of achievement in the wake of dominating another board variety is darn engaging.

From Dissatisfaction to Wellness Enthusiast: My Board Process

For a really long time, my center strength was a disregarded companion. Of course, I'd do an intermittent arrangement of crunches, however how about we be genuine - the outcomes were disappointing. My back would hurt, my structure would endure, and the entire experience felt like an errand. Then, I coincidentally found the universe of boards. From the outset, it was lowering. That apparently straightforward activity left me shaking and scrutinizing my center strength (or scarcity in that department). Be that as it may, with devotion and a little investigation of various board varieties, something mind blowing occurred. My center got more grounded, my back torment evaporated, and a recently discovered certainty sprouted inside me.

<u>**The Center Ensemble: The Muscles Took part in a Board**</u>

A board could appear to be a straightforward hold, however it's a full-body ensemble in camouflage. Here are the central members:

1. **Rectus Abdominis (Abs):** The "six-pack" muscles get a serious exercise during a board, working on their solidarity and definition.

2. **Cross over abdominis:** This profound center muscle assumes a vital part in dependability and stance. Boards connect with this frequently neglected muscle, prompting a more grounded center in general.

3. **Obliques:** These muscles on the sides of your midriff get actuated during boards, further developing center revolution and solidness.

4. **Shoulders:** Boards likewise connect with your shoulders, assisting with further developing stance and forestall wounds.

5. **Glutes and Hamstrings:** To keep a legitimate board position, you really want to connect with your glutes and hamstrings, working these muscles close to your center.

<u>**Building Your Establishment: The Fundamental Board and How to Dominate It**</u>

Before you plunge into the universe of extravagant board varieties, we should nail the fundamental board first. This is a bit by bit guide for fledglings:

- **Get on the Floor:** Begin by lying face down on the floor with your lower arms level on the ground. Your elbows ought to be straightforwardly under your shoulders.
- **Lift Your Body:** Propel yourself up onto your lower arms and toes, shaping a straight line from your head to your heels. Draw in your center by pulling your midsection button towards your spine.
- **Hold it Tight:** Keep up with this situation however long you can serenely hold it. Go for the gold in the first place and slowly increment the hold time as you get more grounded.
- **Center around Structure:** The way into an effective board is legitimate structure. Try not to allow your hips to list or your back curve. Keep your body in an orderly fashion all through the hold.
- **Inhale Simple:** Don't pause your breathing! Make sure to inhale normally all through the activity. Breathe in leisurely through your nose and breathe out through your mouth.

A Vast expanse of Choices: Board Varieties for Each Wellness Level

Now that you've dominated the fundamental board, now is the ideal time to investigate the thrilling universe of varieties! The following are a couple of fledgling well disposed choices to challenge your center and keep things intriguing:

1. **Kneeboard:** This is an extraordinary change for fledglings. Rather than adjusting on your toes, bring down your knees to the ground, keeping your shins and feet level. Center around keeping a straight line from your head to your knees.

2. **Side Board:** This variety focuses on your obliques. Lie on your side with one elbow straightforwardly under your shoulder. Place your feet on top of one another and rise your hips off the ground, shaping a straight line from your head to your feet. Hold however long you can serenely on one side, then change to the opposite side.

3. **High Board:** Assuming you're feeling courageous, attempt the high board. Rather than adjusting on your lower arms, hoist yourself onto

4. **High Board:** Assuming you're feeling brave, attempt the high board. Rather than adjusting on your lower arms, hoist yourself onto your hands, keeping your wrists straightforwardly under your shoulders. This variety requires more chest area strength however offers a more profound center commitment.

5. **Strolling Board:** This unique variety adds a component of trouble and difficulties to your center soundness. Begin in a high board position. Move one hand a couple crawls forward, trailed by the other hand, keeping a straight line with your body all through the development. "Walk" your hands to and fro for a set number of reiterations.

6. **SideBoard with Leg Lift:** Prepared to agree with your position board to a higher level? Whenever you've dominated the fundamental sideboard, take a stab at taking your top leg off the ground. Hold for a couple of moments, then, at that point, bring down your leg and rehash on the opposite side.

7. **Keep in mind:** These are only a couple of models. As you get more grounded, investigate further developed board varieties and find what challenges and invigorates you.

<u>Supportive of Ways to dominate Board Varieties:</u>
- **Warm-up:** In every case warm up prior to beginning any board varieties to set up your muscles and forestall injury.
- **Center around Quality, Not Amount:** It's smarter to hold a board with ideal structure for a more limited length than to forfeit structure for a more extended hold.

- **Movement is Critical:** Don't get deterred on the off chance that you can't hold a board for quite a while at first. Begin with more limited holds and step by step increment the term as you get more grounded.
- **Pay attention to Your Body:** On the off chance that you feel any aggravation, stop the activity and counsel a specialist.

<u>The Board Impact: Past a Solid Center</u>

Board varieties aren't just about building an unshakable center (albeit that is a really magnificent advantage!). Here are a few extra benefits you could insight:

- **Further developed:** Areas of strength for stance muscles add to more readily pose, decreasing back torment and working on your general arrangement.
- **Improved Equilibrium:** Boards challenge your equilibrium and soundness, prompting better coordination and readiness in your everyday exercises.
- **Supported Digestion:** Drawing in numerous muscle bunches during boards can assist with helping your digestion, prompting more productive calorie consumption.
- **Expanded Certainty:** As you ace different board varieties and feel your center getting more grounded, your certainty will normally follow.

You'll move toward your exercises and day to day exercises with a freshly discovered feeling of force and control.

Along these lines, that's essentially it. Board varieties are something beyond an activity - they're an excursion towards a more grounded, more sure you. Embrace the test, investigate the varieties, and feel the mind blowing force of an unshakable center!

Squats: Targeting Lower Body Strength and Core Activation

We should discuss squats, people. They could appear to be a basic activity - simply twist your knees and plunk down, correct? However, trust me, the squat is a stalwart move that merits a position of high standing in any gym routine daily practice. It's not just about etched legs (however those are a decent advantage!). Squats are the establishment for lower body strength, center initiation, and a sensation of strengthening that rises above the exercise center walls.

My excursion with squats wasn't necessarily in every case love at first squat (quip planned). To start with, they felt off-kilter, my structure was sketchy, and can we just look at things objectively for a moment, the consumer was genuine. In any case, with training and a little direction, squats turned out to be something other than an activity - they turned into a similitude forever. They showed me diligence, stretching my boundaries, and the unbelievable things your body can accomplish when you challenge it.

From Cynic to Crouch: Uncovering the Force of the Squat

For quite a long time, I depended on extravagant exercise center machines, dismissing the most essential yet strong development - the squat. Squats felt scary, similar to one side of entry saved for prepared jocks. However at that point, a shrewd coach persuaded me to check them out with legitimate structure. Furthermore, what a disclosure it was! Unexpectedly, squats weren't just about consuming quads - they were a door to a more grounded center, further developed balance, and a recently discovered appreciation for the sheer force of my lower body.

The Ensemble of Solidarity: The Muscles Took part in a Squat

The excellence of the squat lies in its capacity to connect with various muscle bunches all the while. Here is the ensemble playing in your body during an ideal squat:

- **Quadriceps (Quads):** These are the stalwart muscles on the facade of your thighs. Squats work them hard, chiseling and reinforcing them for that conditioned leg look.
- **Hamstrings:** The frequently dismissed muscles on the rear of your thighs get a serious exercise with squats, further developing adaptability and adding capacity to your developments.
- **Glutes:** Squats are a glute-building machine! These muscles add to a chiseled posterior as well as assume a critical part in security and center strength.
- **Center:** Keeping up with legitimate structure during a squat requires center commitment, reinforcing your center, and working on general balance.

Building Your Establishment: A Bit by bit Manual for Dominating the Ideal Squat

Now that you're siphoned (joke expected) about the advantages of squats, we should separate the legitimate structure so you can receive the full benefits. Keep in mind, structure is vital to staying away from injury and augmenting adequacy. This is a bit by bit guide for beginners:

Stand Tall: Begin with your feet shoulder-width separated and your toes pointed somewhat outward (think 10 and 2 o'clock on a clock). Connect with your center by pulling your tummy button towards your spine and envision protracting your spine.

Arrive at Back and Plunk Down: Envision you will plunk down in an imperceptible seat. Pivot at your hips as though you're pushing your glutes back, and curve your knees simultaneously. Place your back straight and your chest raised.

Lower Yourself: Lower yourself down until your thighs are generally lined up with the ground. An effective method for checking profundity is to ensure your knees don't go past your toes.

Propel Yourself Back Up Whenever you've arrived at your squat profundity, connect with your glutes and quads to propel yourself back up to the beginning position. Center around pushing through your heels for a strong lift.

Rehash and Relax: Complete a bunch of squats (go for the gold redundancies to begin) and make sure to inhale all through the development. Breathe in as you lower yourself down, and breathe out as you propel yourself back up.
Supportive of Tips for Fledglings: Excelling at the Squat

Keep Your Back Straight: Abstain from slouching your back during the squat. Keep a tall stance all through the development.

Look Forward: Don't peer down at your feet! Keep your head in accordance with your spine and your look engaged forward.

Try not to Allow Your Knees To collapse As you hunch down, ensure your knees track over your toes and don't buckle internally.

Begin Bodyweight As it were: As a fledgling, center around consummating your structure with bodyweight squats prior to adding loads.

Pay attention to Your Body: Don't propel yourself excessively hard. On the off chance that you feel any aggravation, stop the activity and counsel a specialist.

Past the Nuts and bolts: Squat Varieties to Challenge Yourself - This part could investigate different squat variations like leap squats, Bulgarian split squats, and challis squats, mixing it up and focusing on various muscle gatherings.

The Squat and Your Everyday existence: This segment could examine major areas of strength for how to further develop day to day exercises like climbing steps, conveying food, or playing with your children.

Powering Your Squats: Sustenance for Ideal Execution - This part could give a few essential dietary tips to help your squat exercises and generally speaking wellness objectives.

Just let me know as to whether you'd like me to develop any of these or on the other hand on the off chance that you have an alternate heading as a main priority!

Chapter 9: Maintaining Momentum: Overcoming Challenges and Staying Motivated

Overcoming Challenges and Staying Motivated with Your Kegel Routine

We should discuss a piece of your body that frequently gets covered in mystery - the pelvic floor. It's not precisely evening gathering discussion, but rather trust me, this secret stalwart assumes an essential part in your general prosperity. For my purposes, it was an excursion of self-disclosure, an acknowledgment that went a long way past the room and into the domain of feeling genuinely enabled and in charge. However, can we just be real for a minute, Kegels - the perfect example for pelvic floor works out - aren't generally the simplest propensity to develop.

Perhaps you've heard murmurs regarding Kegels and their alleged advantages. Or on the other hand maybe you're encountering a few pestering issues - urinary spillage, a debilitated center, or even a dunk in charisma. Whatever your justification behind wandering into this domain, welcome on board. We should dig into the universe of reinforcing your pelvic floor muscles with Kegels (and investigate a few other rousing techniques!), and open a universe of advantages that stretch out a long way past what you could at first envision.

From Dissatisfaction to Interest: A Reminder and a Journey for Replies

For a really long time, I disregarded the unobtrusive clues my body was sending. A periodic post-exercise "release," the sensation of a center that wasn't exactly pretty much as solid as it used to be - I dismissed them as minor disturbances. However at that point, things went ahead. An apparently innocuous sniffle transformed into a public humiliation, and the dissatisfaction rose over. Something needed to change.

That is the point at which I coincidentally found the idea of the pelvic floor. This organization of muscles supports your bladder, rectum, and contraceptive organs, going about as an indispensable emotionally supportive network for your whole center. Furthermore, learn to expect the unexpected. Powerless pelvic floor muscles could be the guilty party behind my troubles. Abruptly, those murmurs regarding Kegels didn't appear to be so senseless any longer.

The Murmur Turns into a Thunder: Figuring out the Force of Kegels

Here is the thing about Kegels - they could appear to be basic, however they're inconceivably viable when done accurately. Envision attempting to stop yourself halfway while you're utilizing the washroom - that is the essential Kegel compression. By reinforcing these muscles, you can:

Further develop Bladder Control: Not any more humiliating holes! More grounded pelvic floor muscles can essentially further develop your bladder control, permitting you to take part in exercises without stress.

Improve Center Strength: A solid pelvic floor goes about as an establishment for your center. Further developed center strength means better stance, soundness, and by and large strength.

Support Sexual Capability: For all kinds of people, solid pelvic floor muscles can upgrade sexual delight and capability.

Advance Generally speaking Prosperity: More grounded pelvic floor muscles can affect your whole body, further developing dissemination, supporting post pregnancy recuperation, and in any event, diminishing back torment.

The Restraining of the Internal Pundit: Conquering Normal Kegel Difficulties

Can we just be real for a moment, Kegels can be a test to stay with. Here are a few normal road obstructions and ways to defeat them:

The "Is This In Any Event, Working?" Challenge: these kegel results aren't generally prompt, which can deter. Remain steady, and trust the interaction! You probably won't get results for the time being, yet with devotion, you'll feel the distinction.

The "Wearing Daily schedule out" Challenge: Kegels can feel dreary. Flavor them up! You can do them anyplace, whenever - while cleaning your teeth, sitting in front of the television, or holding up in line. Get inventive!

The "Can't Feel a Thing" Challenge: At times, it's difficult to be aware in the event that you're doing Kegels accurately. Take a stab at doing them while resting with a hand on your stomach. On the off chance that you're getting your pelvic floor muscles accurately, your stomach shouldn't worry.

Building a Kegel Propensity that Endures: Straightforward Procedures for Remaining Roused

Here are a few reasonable tips to assist you with incorporating Kegels flawlessly into your everyday daily practice:

Set Updates: Utilize your telephone's caution or a wellness tracker to remind yourself to do Kegels over the course of the day.

Mate Up: Find a companion who's likewise beginning Kegels and inspire one another.

Keep tabs on Your Development: Keep a basic log or utilize an application to follow your Kegel progress. Seeing improvement can be a strong inspiration.

Reward Yourself: Put forth little objectives and reward yourself for contacting them. Perhaps another exercise outfit or a loosening up absorb the tub!

Past Kegels: An All encompassing Way to deal with Pelvic Floor Wellbeing

Kegels are a fabulous beginning stage, however there's something else to pelvic floor wellbeing besides only one activity.

Solid Propensities: Keeping a sound weight, eating a reasonable eating routine, and remaining hydrated can all add to pelvic floor wellbeing.

Pelvic Floor Stretches: Very much like some other muscle bunch, your pelvic floor muscles can profit from extending. There are delicate stretches you can integrate into your everyday practice to further develop adaptability and blood stream.

Mind-Body Association: Stress can negatively affect your pelvic floor wellbeing. Rehearses like yoga, contemplation, and profound breathing can assist with overseeing pressure and work on in general prosperity.

Proficient Assistance: Assuming you're encountering tenacious issues like urinary incontinence or pelvic agony, go ahead and proficient assistance. An actual advisor spend significant time in pelvic floor wellbeing can make a customized program to address your particular necessities.

Keep in mind, you are in good company! Pelvic floor issues are extraordinarily normal, and there's no disgrace in looking for help. By assuming responsibility for your pelvic floor wellbeing, you're putting resources into your general prosperity and enabling yourself to carry on with a daily existence liberated from impediments.

All in all, would you say you are prepared to release the force of your pelvic floor? With a touch of devotion and the right methodology, you can overcome those murmurs and experience the fantastic advantages of areas of strength for a solid pelvic floor.

Celebrating Progress and Recognizing Achievements

We as a whole pursue that inclination - the surge of triumph, the confetti shower of progress. It's the summit of long evenings, constant exertion, and the steady conviction that we can accomplish our objectives. However, here's reality, my companions: the way to accomplishment is seldom a straight shot to the champagne toast. It's more similar to a winding street loaded up with diversions, potholes, and minutes where the end goal appears to subside into the distance.

This is where the specialty of celebrating progress comes in. It's tied in with recognizing the little triumphs, the gradual advances that prepare for the fantastic finale. Since we can just be real for a minute, in the event that we just celebrate coming to the mountain ridge, we pass up the whole stunning excursion.

From Debilitation to Disclosure: A Missed Achievement and a Flash of Progress

Some time ago I was fixated on the objective, heedless to the meaning of the excursion. I was preparing for a long distance race, focused on crossing the end goal that the day to day miles obscured into a dreary trudge. Each missed speed target felt like an individual disappointment, a devastating catastrophe for my spirit. It was only after I hit an especially beating level that something moved down. Conversing with an individual sprinter, a carefully prepared long distance runner with a gleam in his expression, caused me to acknowledge I was overlooking the main issue completely. He wasn't simply commending the race day - he was delighting in each vanquished slope, each private best, every dawn that welcomed him on his preparation runs.

The Force of the "Small scale Me" Festivities: Powering Your Excursion

That discussion was a defining moment. I began recognizing the little triumphs - the additional mile I drove myself to run, whenever I first aced that slope run, the sheer delight of putting on my running shoes and venturing out the entryway. These "scaled down me" festivities weren't tied in with gloating privileges - they were tied in with recognizing my work, filling my natural inspiration, and reminding myself why I left on this excursion in any case.

The Orchestra of Self-Appreciation: Advantages of Observing Advancement

Here is the lovely thing about celebrating progress: it goes past a straightforward mental congratulatory gesture. It significantly affects your whole process:

Helped Inspiration: Recognizing your achievements, regardless of how little, powers your inspiration to continue onward. An injection of encouraging feedback reminds you why you began and keeps you pushing forward.

Upgraded Certainty: Celebrating progress constructs your certainty. As you see yourself accomplishing, even the more modest objectives, you foster a confidence in your own capacities, engaging you to handle greater difficulties.

Further developed Determination: The way to accomplishment is seldom smooth. Misfortunes are unavoidable. In any case, when you celebrate progress, you develop a feeling of flexibility. You figure out how to see mishaps as brief barricades, not unrealistic walls.

More prominent Happiness: Praising the excursion makes the whole cycle more pleasant. It moves your concentration from the far off finish line to the current second, permitting you to enjoy the experience and value the development you're encountering.

Tracking down Your Festival Language: Customized Ways Of recognizing Your Successes

There's no one size-fits-all way to deal with celebrating progress. The key is to find what impacts you, what lights a flash of happiness, and fills your inspiration. The following are a couple of thoughts to kick you off let's go:

The Diary Passage: Require a couple of moments toward the finish of every day to consider your advancement. Write down your triumphs, enormous or little, to make an individual log of your accomplishments.

The Prize Custom: Put forth little objectives and reward yourself for contacting them. It very well may be anything from a loosening up bubble shower to enjoying your number one sound treat.

The Appreciation Custom: Offer thanks for your achievements. Require a second to see the value in your work, your strength, and your obligation to development.

The Representation Festivity: Carve out opportunity to envision yourself accomplishing your definitive objective. Permit yourself to feel the feelings of accomplishment, and utilize that inclination to move you forward.

The Last Lap: Observing Advancement is a Deep rooted Excursion

Celebrating progress isn't just about accomplishing a particular objective - it's a long lasting practice. It's tied in with developing an appreciation for the excursion, for the work we put in, and for the individual we become en route. Thus, my companions, we should raise a figurative glass to each forward-moving step, each challenge vanquished, each triumph - huge or little. Since at the end of the day, the excursion of self-revelation, of development, and of turning into our best selves that genuinely merits the thunderous applause

Incorporating Kegel Activities into Your Regular routine for Long haul Advantages

We should discuss a distinct advantage, a secret hero in the domain of wellbeing and prosperity - the pelvic floor. An organization of muscles probably won't get a great deal of evening gathering discussion, yet trust me, it assumes an essential part in your general feeling of control and certainty. As far as I might be concerned, it was an excursion of self-revelation, an acknowledgment that went a long ways past actual advantages. It was tied in with assuming responsibility and putting resources into my drawn out wellbeing.

However, can we just be real, Kegels, the perfect example for pelvic floor works out, aren't generally the simplest propensity to develop. They can feel off-kilter, the outcomes could appear to be subtle, and squeezing them into a bustling life can be a test. However, stop and think for a minute - the advantages areas of strength for of floor muscles are irrefutable, and the uplifting news is, that incorporating Kegels into your regular routine doesn't need to be a task. With a touch of imagination and a sprinkle of self-empathy, you can open a universe of advantages that reach out a long way past what you could at first envision.

From Disappointment to Opportunity: A Reminder and the Force of Consistency

For a really long time, I overlooked the unobtrusive signs - a periodic "spill" after a wheeze, the sensation of a center that wasn't exactly pretty much as solid as it used to be. I forgot about them as minor disturbances. However at that point, something moved. The dissatisfaction rose over, and I realized I needed to assume command. That is the point at which I coincidentally found the idea of the pelvic floor. These secret muscles, similar to an ensemble guide, coordinate bladder control, sexual capability, and event center dependability.

The disclosure was basic at this point significant - by reinforcing these muscles, I could recover a feeling of opportunity and certainty. Certainly, Kegels could appear to be a murmur calm activity, however with consistency, they could turn into a thunder of strengthening.

The Orchestra Inside: Understanding the Advantages Areas of strength for of Floor Muscles

Here is the wizardry of Kegels - they're straightforward yet unimaginably viable when done accurately. Envision attempting to stop yourself halfway while you're utilizing the washroom - that is the essential Kegel withdrawal. By reinforcing these muscles, you can open a universe of advantages, including:

Resolute Certainty: No more breaks or stresses! More grounded pelvic floor muscles mean a recently discovered feeling of trust in all that you do, from high-influence exercises to unconstrained undertakings.

A More grounded Center: The pelvic floor behaves like an establishment for your center. Further developed center strength implies better stance, expanded solidness, and generally speaking strength for all your everyday exercises.

Upgraded Closeness: For all kinds of people, solid pelvic floor muscles can prompt a more charming and satisfying personal life.

Deep rooted: Major areas of strength for venture floor muscles can help you all through your life, supporting post pregnancy recuperation, lessening back torment, and advancing generally speaking prosperity.

Past the Fundamentals: Innovative Systems for Coordinating Kegels into Your Day

Can we just look at things objectively for a minute, customary work-out schedules can feel dreary. However,

Kegels are unique - they're a clear-cut advantage you can employ carefully over the course of your day. Here are an inventive ways of coordinating Kegels consistently into your life:

The Morning Lift: Begin your day with a bunch of Kegels while cleaning your teeth. It's a fast and simple method for establishing the vibe for a sure day.

The Worker Crush: Trapped in rush hour gridlock? Flip around that grimace (and fortify your pelvic floor!) with a couple watchful Kegels while you pause.

The Lift Commitment: Those short lift rides are the ideal chance for a speedy arrangement of Kegels. Nobody will be the most astute, and your pelvic floor will be much obliged.

The Performing various tasks Expert: Consolidate Kegels with different exercises you as of now do. Hold them while holding up in line, taking care of tasks, or in any event, staring at the television.

The Kegel Challenge: Make it fun! Challenge yourself to do a specific number of Kegels over the course of the day and prize yourself for arriving at your objectives.

<u>**Building a Kegel Propensity that Endures: The Force of Self-Empathy**</u>

Here is the key - be thoughtful to yourself. Building a Kegel propensity takes time and consistency. Try not to get deterred on the off chance that you miss a meeting or two. Simply get yourself and refocus. Here are a few extra tips for long haul achievement:

Keep tabs on Your Development: Utilize a basic log or application to follow your Kegel progress. Seeing improvement, regardless of how little, can be a strong inspiration.

Chapter 10: The Power Within: Conclusion and Taking Charge of Your Health

We've arrived at the finish of this excursion together, haven't we? An excursion that wasn't just about actual wellbeing, yet about self-revelation, strengthening, and recovering control. Maybe you began perusing these pages feeling lost, overpowered by the apparently unending stream of wellbeing data and clashing guidance. Perhaps you held onto questions about your capacity to accomplish your objectives, a voice murmuring that assuming responsibility for your wellbeing was excessively overwhelming, excessively convoluted.

In any case, here's reality I've come to trust through my own encounters: the ability to change your wellbeing exists in you. There's actually no need to focus on pursuing some unreachable ideal or capitulating to the trend eats less carbs. It's tied in with settling on cognizant decisions, slowly and carefully, that line up with your qualities and engage you to feel your best.

<u>From Doubter to Self-Supporter: My Change</u>

Thinking back, I can pinpoint the second everything moved. It was anything but an emotional revelation, however a steady collection of little triumphs. Whenever I first finished a bunch of activities without feeling like I planned to fall. The acknowledgment that a good feast could be both flavorful and feeding. The freshly discovered certainty that blossomed from focusing on my prosperity. These minutes, hung together, shaped a strong story: I was certainly not an uninvolved traveler on the wellbeing venture; I was the driver, graphing the course and going with cognizant decisions that energized my change.

<u>The Excursion Proceeds: Difficulties and Mishaps Are Inescapable</u>

This isn't to say the street has been smooth. There were (and will be) days when inspiration melted away, desires snuck in, and the compulsion to return to old propensities posed a potential threat. In any case, here's the key: mishaps don't characterize you. They're just diversions on your wellbeing process, chances to learn, change, and commit once again to your objectives. The significant thing is to get yourself, dust yourself off, and continue to push ahead.

Building a Maintainable Way of life, Not an Intensive lesson

Quite possibly the main example I've learned is that enduring change requires an economical way of life, not a compressed lesson in hardship. It's tied in with finding sound propensities you can coordinate into your day to day daily practice, not tied in with pursuing convenient solutions. It's tied in with paying attention to your body's exceptional necessities and respecting them. Every so often, a delicate yoga meeting may be all you want. On different days, a focused energy exercise may be your best pressure reliever. The key is to embrace adaptability and find what turns out best for you.

The Far reaching influence: How Your Responsibility Rouses Others

The groundbreaking force of assuming responsibility for your wellbeing doesn't stop at you. It has a far reaching influence, rousing people around you. Perhaps it's your accomplice going along with you for a walk, a companion requesting solid recipe proposals, or your kid seeing your commitment to taking care of oneself. By focusing on your prosperity, you're sending a strong message - that wellbeing is an excursion worth taking, and that assuming command over your decisions can prompt a more joyful, more engaged life.

A Last Word: Embrace the Excursion, Praise the Triumphs

As you close this part and leave on your own wellbeing process, recall this: it's a long distance race, not a run. There will be highs and lows, snapshots of uncertainty, and snapshots of win. In any case, the ability to make enduring change exists in you. Embrace the excursion, commend the triumphs (of all shapes and sizes!), and above all, believe constantly in your capacity to be the best, most joyful variant of yourself.

This isn't farewell, but instead a "see you on the way." Continue pushing ahead, continue learning, and continue to assume responsibility for your unbelievable power inside.

Day	Positions	Sets	Rep/Hold Seconds	Notes
1				
2				
3				
4				
5				
6				
7				
8				
9				
10				
11				

KEGEL EXERCISE CHART

Day	Positions	Sets	Rep/Hold Seconds	Notes
1				
2				
3				
4				
5				
6				
7				
8				
9				
10				
11				

KEGEL EXERCISE CHART

Day	Positions	Sets	Rep/Hold Seconds	Notes
1				
2				
3				
4				
5				
6				
7				
8				
9				
10				
11				

KEGEL EXERCISE CHART

Day	Positions	Sets	Rep/Hold Seconds	Notes
1				
2				
3				
4				
5				
6				
7				
8				
9				
10				
11				

KEGEL EXERCISE CHART

Day	Positions	Sets	Rep/Hold Seconds	Notes
1				
2				
3				
4				
5				
6				
7				
8				
9				
10				
11				

KEGEL EXERCISE CHART

Day	Positions	Sets	Rep/Hold Seconds	Notes
1				
2				
3				
4				
5				
6				
7				
8				
9				
10				
11				

KEGEL EXERCISE CHART

Day	Positions	Sets	Rep/Hold Seconds	Notes
1				
2				
3				
4				
5				
6				
7				
8				
9				
10				
11				

KEGEL EXERCISE CHART

Day	Positions	Sets	Rep/Hold Seconds	Notes
1				
2				
3				
4				
5				
6				
7				
8				
9				
10				
11				

KEGEL EXERCISE CHART

Day	Positions	Sets	Rep/Hold Seconds	Notes
1				
2				
3				
4				
5				
6				
7				
8				
9				
10				
11				

KEGEL EXERCISE CHART

Day	Positions	Sets	Rep/Hold Seconds	Notes
1				
2				
3				
4				
5				
6				
7				
8				
9				
10				
11				

KEGEL EXERCISE CHART

Day	Morning section (Sets/Reps/Hold)	Afternoon Section Sets/Reps/Hold	Evening Section Sets/Reps/Hold	Note
Monday				
Tuesday				
Wednesday				
Thursday				
Friday				
Saturday				
Sunday				

kegel exercise tracker

Day	Morning section (Sets/Reps/Hold)	Afternoon Section Sets/Reps/Hold	Evening Section Sets/Reps/Hold	Note
Monday				
Tuesday				
Wednesday				
Thursday				
Friday				
Saturday				
Sunday				

kegel exercise tracker

Day	Morning section (Sets/Reps/Hold	Afternoon Section Sets/Reps/Hold	Evening Section Sets/Reps/Hold	Note
Monday				
Tuesday				
Wednesday				
Thursday				
Friday				
Saturday				
Sunday				

kegel exercise tracker

Day	Morning section (Sets/Reps/Hold)	Afternoon Section Sets/Reps/Hold	Evening Section Sets/Reps/Hold	Note
Monday				
Tuesday				
Wednesday				
Thursday				
Friday				
Saturday				
Sunday				

kegel exercise tracker

Day	Morning section (Sets/Reps/Hold	Afternoon Section Sets/Reps/Hold	Evening Section Sets/Reps/Hold	Note
Monday				
Tuesday				
Wednesday				
Thursday				
Friday				
Saturday				
Sunday				

kegel exercise tracker

Day	Morning section (Sets/Reps/Hold	Afternoon Section Sets/Reps/Hold	Evening Section Sets/Reps/Hold	Note
Monday				
Tuesday				
Wednesday				
Thursday				
Friday				
Saturday				
Sunday				

kegel exercise tracker

Day	Morning section (Sets/Reps/Hold	Afternoon Section Sets/Reps/Hold	Evening Section Sets/Reps/Hold	Note
Monday				
Tuesday				
Wednesday				
Thursday				
Friday				
Saturday				
Sunday				

kegel exercise tracker

Day	Morning section (Sets/Reps/Hold	Afternoon Section Sets/Reps/Hold	Evening Section Sets/Reps/Hold	Note
Monday				
Tuesday				
Wednesday				
Thursday				
Friday				
Saturday				
Sunday				

kegel exercise tracker

Day	Morning section (Sets/Reps/Hold	Afternoon Section Sets/Reps/Hold	Evening Section Sets/Reps/Hold	Note
Monday				
Tuesday				
Wednesday				
Thursday				
Friday				
Saturday				
Sunday				

kegel exercise tracker

Day	Morning section (Sets/Reps/Hold	Afternoon Section Sets/Reps/Hold	Evening Section Sets/Reps/Hold	Note
Monday				
Tuesday				
Wednesday				
Thursday				
Friday				
Saturday				
Sunday				

kegel exercise tracker

9 798324 588021